THE ANXIOUS PERSON'S GUIDE
TO NON-MONOGAMY

of related interest

How to Understand Your Sexuality
A Practical Guide for Exploring Who You Are
Meg-John Barker and Alex Iantaffi
Illustrated by Jules Scheele
ISBN 978 1 78775 618 2
eISBN 978 1 78775 619 9

Queer Sex
A Trans and Non-Binary Guide to Intimacy, Pleasure and Relationships
Juno Roche
ISBN 978 1 78592 406 4
eISBN 978 1 78450 770 1

Life Isn't Binary
On Being Both, Beyond, and In-Between
Meg-John Barker and Alex Iantaffi
ISBN 978 1 78592 479 8
eISBN 978 1 78450 864 7

The A–Z of Gender and Sexuality
From Ace to Ze
Morgan Lev Edward Holleb
ISBN 978 1 78592 342 5
eISBN 978 1 78450 663 6

Coming Out Stories
Personal Experiences of Coming Out from Across the LGBTQ+ Spectrum
Edited by Emma Goswell and Sam Walker
ISBN 978 1 78775 495 9
eISBN 978 1 78775 496 6

THE ANXIOUS PERSON'S GUIDE TO NON-MONOGAMY

Your Guide to Open Relationships, Polyamory and Letting Go

LOLA PHOENIX

Foreword by
Kathy G. Slaughter, LCSW

Jessica Kingsley Publishers
London and Philadelphia

First published in Great Britain in 2022 by Jessica Kingsley Publishers
An imprint of Hodder & Stoughton Ltd
An Hachette Company

1

Trigger Warning: This book mentions sexual
abuse, trauma, anxiety and depression.

A CIP catalogue record for this title is available from
the British Library and the Library of Congress

ISBN 978 1 83997 213 3
eISBN 978 1 83997 214 0

Printed and bound in the United States by Integrated Books International

Jessica Kingsley Publishers' policy is to use papers that are natural,
renewable and recyclable products and made from wood grown in
sustainable forests. The logging and manufacturing processes are expected
to conform to the environmental regulations of the country of origin.

Jessica Kingsley Publishers
Carmelite House
50 Victoria Embankment
London EC4Y 0DZ

www.jkp.com

Contents

Foreword

Years ago, as I began my journey into polyamory and working with polyamorous clients, I found most of the 'starter' books available inadequate. While I loved the inspiration contained in *The Ethical Slut*, and I believe *Opening Up*, by Tristan Taormino, might be the best beginner's manual out there, it was clear to me these books were missing an important perspective.

This perspective was an understanding of trauma, queer identities and disability. Developmental trauma – being abused as a child – was my first professional specialty. As a clinical social worker, I've worked with hundreds of people impacted by trauma early in their lives. I'm also a childhood trauma survivor myself. And I've been the anonymous relationship therapist reviewing Lola's work for the past several years.

Now, after years working with polyamorous clients, I've noticed that jumping into a non-monogamous relationship style can bring old pain and anxiety screaming to the surface. Often my clients worry that they're not 'cut out' for polyamory because their emotional reactions are so intense. And when I looked at the available resources for support, I understood where this fear came from.

It's also why I so highly value Lola Phoenix and their work. In my early days, when my own insecurities threatened to torpedo my polyamorous ambitions, their posts reflected my experience more accurately than any other polyam advice out there. Lola understood the significance of emotions, the ways they deserve to be honored and how to feel your feelings.

Much of the mainstream polyam advice and the perspectives of many polyam communities that I belong to make emotions seem irrational, irrelevant and barriers to this relationship style. And it's true, emotional uproar does impact our interpersonal relationships in ways that can blow a polycule apart. However, treating emotions as a hindrance, personal failing or something that can be discarded is the wrong approach.

I like to think of emotions as embodied thoughts. What we call anger or sadness is our mind's attempt to make sense of how the body feels. And in my experience, when we try to avoid hearing what our body wants to tell us, those emotions just get stronger and stronger until we do pause and acknowledge them. When emotions get really intense, it can also increase our sense of urgency that something must be done to make these feelings go away, right now!

And maybe that's true. One of Lola's gifts is understanding how a situation can feel bad because it *is* bad. One of your partners might genuinely be mistreating you. And sometimes feelings are related to something else from our past, not the way one of our partners is behaving. In order to sort all that out and decide how you want to proceed you must feel the feelings first. Only by becoming acquainted with them can you find the right solution for you.

After recommending Lola's column and podcast for years, I am delighted to have their perspective captured in this book. Jumping into an open relationship can be a bit like jumping off a cliff. You likely spent years thinking about your future romantic relationship before you started dating. And our mono-centric culture offers plenty of resources, role models and ideas about what romantic relationships should look like. When you start practicing non-monogamy, those resources are substantially less. The time you've spent learning and thinking about what type of open relationship you want is less. And so, it can be very difficult to discern what's going on in your new non-mono relationship.

So, we turn to books and others who are practicing this lovestyle for guidance. And the advice you will encounter is all over the place. You'll find folks who insist that all approaches to non-monogamy are equally valid, and you'll find folks who insist that a particular style is the only way to go. It can be incredibly hard to find your way and discover what you want and what works for you and your partners.

Lola's book will support you in *your* path as an individual. Reading their work is like talking to a pragmatic, caring non-judgmental BFF who's been there. Their own experience gives them a unique perspective, and they will give you permission to honor your feelings and your desires. The first section in particular offers guidance on how to turn inside and build your own foundation.

The second section addresses the conflicting and strong opinions you'll find in the literature and in polyam communities. It's so beneficial to explore and unpack jealousy from a non-judgmental place, to understand the limits of communities run by volunteers, and to begin to understand how power dynamics can impact you and your chosen family.

The middle section dives deeper into the nitty-gritty of the logistics of being in multiple relationships at once, which I love, because so many polyam basics authors can skip over the emotions that can be revealed when your week needs to include multiple date nights. Google Calendar can keep you sane, but it can't promise nobody's feelings get hurt.

Finally, Lola takes the time to preview some of the emotions you'll feel when you actually start doing this thing. Many people I know read all the polyamory material and felt super equipped to start their adventure, and then...rubber meets the road. And it's not what they expect. No matter how firmly you intellectually believe non-monogamy is for you, that doesn't guarantee your emotions will be on the same page. Knowing what you may feel will definitely help you the first time you're dealing with your partner falling in love with someone else!

It's been an honor to oversee and edit Lola's work, including this book. You're holding a real treat and a valuable resource in your hands right now. I believe you will find their perspective as valuable as I did. Enjoy!

Kathy G. Slaughter, LCSW
Founder of Soaring Heart Center in Indianapolis, Indiana, USA
Trauma & Sexuality Therapist

Introduction

I came to non-monogamy by way of sex-positive communities when I was trying to reconnect with my body and sexuality after finally really coming to terms with the sexual abuse I'd been through as a child. A lot of what sex-positive communities did was encourage questioning the things society had taught me about sex, which then led to questioning the assumptions society had about monogamy.

Originally, when I wanted children, I thought non-monogamy was a great way to create an environment where a child would experience multiple caregivers who would be there to provide for them, especially given my disability could potentially lead me into needing more care myself when I got older. My interest was purely practical, rather than necessarily rooted in an internal desire to love more than one person or a strong attraction to more than one person.

It's always been a habit of mine to do as much research as possible about something that I have an interest in and polyamory was no exception. I read a lot of advice and did my best to prepare for what I thought would be much easier for me if I just read the information I needed to read. A lot of it made logical sense and seemed fairly straightforward and when I entered into 'the community' where I was, I felt like I had a lot of support and a lot of people who had 'experience' whom I could trust. The first couple of times the advice I gathered didn't work, I thought it was my fault.

So much of what I learned was encouraging distrust of my own judgement, a reinforcement of the same denial I had of my own emotions my entire life and a reinforcement of the idea that, by being on the asexual spectrum, my lack of interest in casual sex wasn't part of a valid expression of sexuality but evidence that I needed to overcome the shackles of a puritanical society. Nothing I learned fostered a closer connection to my own emotions, taught me how to calm my nervous system or helped me negotiate boundaries.

It's no surprise then that my first experiences with polyamory were extremely sketchy and I only managed to escape them by reading literature about abusive relationships and abusive patterns, specifically the book *Why Does He Do That?* by Lundy Bancroft, which I frequently recommend. I wouldn't until much later learn that my negative emotions weren't inherently a sign of my own insecurity. I grew frustrated with problems I and others had that I constantly saw crop up that weren't really talked about. I felt like so much of what polyamory advice offered me either didn't address mental health or just didn't work for someone who had the anxiety or the experiences I had growing up. So I did what I usually do when I have thoughts: I wrote them down.

I started writing articles about polyamory in 2015 and then, after writing a few more and participating in a few online polyamory communities, I was directly asked for advice. I had enjoyed giving advice so much that I decided to try to write an advice column and Non-Monogamy Help was born in January 2017. Two years later, I decided to start a podcast version and I have been giving advice in the column and on the podcast since then.

I found that I wasn't the only one that felt that way and, even though I received a lot of pushback from people, I received more encouragement from other people who felt like they had been alone in their feelings too. Since I began putting 'polyamorous' or 'non-monogamous' on my dating bios over a decade ago, my 'practice' has shifted, especially after learning more about anarchist perspectives, towards something like relationship anarchy and away from hierarchies, but with a heavy emphasis on seeing how people behave to see what they practise, rather than just trusting a label.

Polyamory for me is a choice, though I recognize and respect that some people do not feel that way. For me, it being a choice doesn't make it less valid. Many aspects of my life are choices that I make that better my mental health and that would lead to something worse if I didn't make that choice. Instead of being someone who has romantic or sexual feelings frequently, for me, what led me to polyamory was that, because I am so rarely interested in people, I want the chance to pursue that if and when the stars rightly align (and they're also interested in me). Monogamy is a choice I could make, but not one I have wanted to make any time soon.

After ten years of 'practice' and multiple columns and podcasts, I do not think I am an expert. I do not think my relationship style is on a higher level than others. I dislike any kind of discourse that, even accidentally, pits polyamory as a superior choice for everyone over monogamy. I still have anxiety. I've felt jealousy and didn't just 'get over it' because it made sense for me to be jealous in those time periods or sometimes it didn't. Ultimately, the only person who can decide if polyamory or non-monogamy is right for you is you, not me, even with a decade of what could loosely be called 'experience'.

But I hope what this book will bring you is some comfort that the struggles you're facing are not ones you're facing alone. Hopefully this can give you some understanding if you have a partner who is struggling with some of the same things I have struggled and do struggle with. As much as some believe human beings are apex predators who thrive on rugged individualism, we're ultimately social animals and feeling alone in our pain makes that pain much harder to cope with. You're not alone.

This book is divided into sections designed for someone who is at the beginning of their interest in non-monogamy, though it could still work for someone who has been non-monogamous for years. We'll start with what I think you'll need to begin, which includes a section on how to find an anchor, to figure out a personal reasoning for wanting to pursue non-monogamy, how to challenge your fears effectively, and actualizing your needs and practising self-compassion.

The next section, on what you will hear and read, discusses topics you'll approach in most polyamory media including jealousy, independence, the issues you may have with communities and the crab in bucket mentalities you may end up coming across. We'll then explore the physicalities of non-monogamy in the section on what you will do, including scheduling your time, planning for emergencies, checking in and working through boundary negotiation. Finally, the last section on what you'll feel includes information about how to prepare for unexpected bumps, metamour complications, as well as struggles with comparison and definitions of success.

With this book, I wanted to do more than repeat some of the advice I have given in the podcast and column. I've expanded on it here, but I've also decided to add more. After each section, there will be a series of challenges you can complete on your own or with a partner. These aren't designed to solve or address every single problem but may help create clarity out of some of the confusing aspects of starting off in non-monogamy. I wanted this not to be just another book to read, but something you can do and put into actual practice.

Maybe in ten more years, I will be able to teach everyone how to reach a state where you never experience jealousy, only experience compersion, never have any problems, and your biggest problem is wrangling with Google Calendar. Maybe in ten more years, I'll have figured out the recipe for a truly perfect polyamory that will convince even the staunchest monogamist to come over to this side.

But, somehow, I doubt it.

As I say in the column and on the podcast, I hope this helps and good luck.

Glossary

compersion – sometimes described as 'the opposite of jealousy', compersion is a feeling of joy or happiness in witnessing or hearing about a partner's attraction or love for another person and/or relationship successes or wins. Example: When Martha told me about how well her date went, I felt so much compersion!

don't ask, don't tell/DADT – A term coined from the US approach towards homosexuality within the military. Within polyamorous communities it describes a relationship style involving a couple where either one or both members of the couple are allowed to have sexual relationships outside of the prioritized couple and have a strict policy of not telling each other any details about other relationships and completely hiding it so that the other partner would never know.

hard limit – A completely non-negotiable thing. Example: While I'm okay with occasional visits from nieces or nephews, living with kids over a two-week period is a hard limit.

hinge – This describes an individual who is effectively in the 'middle' of two different partners who do not date.

kitchen table polyamory – A term coined by Megan Bhatia, Marty Bhatia and Kyle Henry in their Amory podcast which describes a situation where partners and metamours regularly communicate, get along with and befriend each other as one would a family.

metamour – A person whom your partner dates who is not your partner. Example: Tony is my partner. Tony dates Adam. I don't date Adam. Adam is my metamour.

monogamish – A term describing individuals who feel like they don't fit within the boundaries of monogamy or polyamory or may practise monogamy usually but occasionally open their relationship for sexual events, threesomes, orgies, etc.

monogamy – A relationship practice where two individuals promise romantic and sexual exclusivity to each other.

new relationship energy/NRE – A term describing the rush of energy and excitement that accompanies a new and budding relationship.

one penis policy/OPP – A rule implemented usually upon cis women by a cis male partner where the woman is not allowed to have other male partners. OPP does not usually include any nuanced definitions of where women with penises, men with vaginas, intersex people or non-binary people with any genitalia fall into the policy.

open relationship – An umbrella term describing any relationship between a couple which does not involve sexual or romantic fidelity.

parallel polyamory – A style of polyamory where partners and metamours may know about each other but do not intentionally meet up or communicate unless necessary.

polycule – A term describing not just one relationship structure but also the metamours involved as well.

polyfidelity – A term describing a polyamorous relationship of any number of individuals where the individuals only have sexual or romantic relationships with the individuals within the polyamorous relationship.

quad – Four individuals in a relationship with each other.

relationship anarchy – a term coined by Andie Nordgren in the essay 'The short instructional manifesto for relationship anarchy'. This is a way of applying anarchist principles to relationships focusing on anti-hierarchy, respect of individual autonomy and compassion.

solo polyamory – An individual who chooses to not cohabitate with other partners.

swinging – A practice of open relationships where, usually a couple, attends events or is involved in a community where partner swapping, threesomes or orgies are allowed. Usually this happens at specific regulated events and is only a sexual rather than a romantic practice.

triad – Three individuals in a relationship with each other.

unicorn hunters/unicorn hunting – A term with origins in the swinger community. Unicorn hunters are usually a couple that is a cis heterosexual man and a cis bisexual woman looking for another bisexual woman, or 'third', for a closed triad who has no other partners and who will not only love both individuals in the couple 'equally' but will also likely be 'sacrificed' or dumped to save the original couple if jealousy or anything else arises.

vee – A polyamorous relationship structure composed of a hinge and two of the hinge's partners.

veto – A policy whereby, usually in a couple group, a member of the group can request that their partner dump someone that they are dating, or they get to 'veto' metamours.

What Will You Need?

∞

There are quite a few books that are recommended for people interested in polyamory and non-monogamy. One of the reasons why I started to write articles about non-monogamy and eventually to give advice was because I felt like everything that I had read had either not prepared me properly for the challenges I had or had actively undermined my efforts to try and cope with the shift from monogamy to non-monogamy.

This isn't to say that, had I been better prepared, I would have been able to avoid some of the emotional difficulties that polyamory caused me. I think the biggest and first mistake people make is trying to avoid feeling bad or avoid difficult emotions that non-monogamy can bring when they enter into it. But it's to say that, if I had the tools that I'm about to hopefully impart to you, coping would have been far easier.

This first chapter covers what you may need in starting out.

FIND YOUR ANCHOR

Polyamory is not monogamy with an upgrade. It is a different way of living. If a couple expecting a child believed that having that child wouldn't change the way they lived day to day, we'd consider that unrealistic. Likewise, it is unrealistic to believe that switching from monogamy to polyamory will not change the way you live your day-to-day life in relationships. It may not at first seem all that different, but things will definitely change.

If you're going to change the way you live your day-to-day life, especially in a world that has given you little to no support in reckoning that way of life, you're going to need something to hold onto or, ultimately, a very good reason why you've decided to make that change that you can reflect on when times are hard to help you cope.

I call it an **anchor** and the most important thing about an anchor when it comes to polyamory is that it has to be about you. Your reason for trying polyamory or non-monogamy has to be a benefit or something that it brings to you and you alone because it's meant to be something solid you can rely on. If you base it on someone else, preserving a monogamous relationship or a set of circumstances that you can't control, it may not work well in the long run.

If your best friend came to you and expressed wanting to have a child to keep their partner faithful or engaged in their relationship, you would, hopefully, advise that this isn't a good decision. This is because having a child can't change the whims of a partner, though it may be an activity that could increase bonding between two parents and seem, on the surface, like it is changing the behaviour of the other person.

When many people are introduced to polyamory or non-monogamy, they are usually already in a monogamous relationship and their partner comes to them wanting to try it or feeling this is the way they were for a long time and now they feel monogamy can't work for them. And when this happens, many people will only choose to try polyamory or non-monogamy to keep their partner in their life and avoid a breakup – not for any other reason.

There are also people who come to polyamory or non-monogamy because they are interested in someone who is polyamorous or non-monogamous themselves. It can be incredibly tempting to want to choose polyamory in that case so that you can have a relationship you want to have, especially if you're caught up in the excitement of it.

But, as I mentioned before, polyamory is not monogamy with an upgrade. If you agree to a polyamorous or non-monogamous relationship style, you are fundamentally agreeing that your partner will not spend all of their available time with you. I believe some monogamous relationships where one of the people has a time-intensive career or hobby may also have a similar setup – but those are not monogamous relationships that all monogamous people want to be in.

Therefore, agreeing to polyamory to keep the relationship you have – which is monogamous – alive and as it currently exists is like agreeing to a long-distance relationship to keep an in-person relationship going in an in-person way. It will not work if you believe your relationship will not fundamentally change.

NOTE YOUR REASONING

If you are only coming to non-monogamy because your partner wants to try it and you suspect, even if they smile and carry on, they may break up with you if you *don't* try it, it might be difficult to find any benefit to non-monogamy that isn't saving the relationship. That might just be what is primarily motivating you to make it work.

There's only so much I think you can do to avoid that. And I won't lie, keeping your relationship, especially if you have spent a long time fostering it, can be a pretty decent motivator to do all sorts of things, but what's important is that you understand that the fundamentals of your relationship *will* change, if not right away than eventually.

Your reasoning can't be the wool that you pull over your eyes. Many people, myself included, feel perfectly comfortable with the *thought* of non-monogamy but feel very differently when the reality comes knocking on their door. That's when your anchors will be truly tested. Having a personal reason can be something *more* to cling on to.

Finding a personal reason can be difficult, especially when your relationship is threatened, but if you take a moment to consider the way monogamy has been positioned into your life, most of the time you *can* find a reason to give non-monogamy a try. Monogamy is a socially encouraged norm for many people and they don't often think about their motivations for choosing it. We spend our entire lives, even as children, with the concept of monogamy as a destination and imagining the various ways our lives will be moulded around it.

Pulling that rug out from under us causes anxiety – and that's not even the anxiety that naturally comes from fearing the loss of a relationship. If you consider how long you've spent in your life pondering marriage, playing 'House' and all sorts of other cultural scripts your brain has downloaded through films, television and all of the media you've consumed, you're basically trying to make up for many, many years of thinking very quickly. It's a lot.

Here are some basic assumptions society has passed onto you that you can challenge in order to find a personal reason to explore non-monogamy:

Romantic love is the most important love

While it's not necessarily something a lot of people talk about going through, many people have experienced a situation where their friend has started a relationship and, suddenly, they fall off the face of the Earth. They stop prioritizing their friendships because they see romantic relationships as more important.

We're furthermore encouraged to think this way in how we talk about romance. Going from a friendship to a romantic relationship is considered 'more than friends' and the reverse is considered being 'just friends'. Some of these issues are complicated by the fact that close friendships between men are often discouraged, people question whether men and women can 'really be friends' and queer relationships are often seen as platonic friendships or forced to be considered socially as friendships in places where it's unsafe to be out.

And yet, many of us have had very close friendships that meant a lot to us. When I've personally talked about the pain of a friendship breakup and how it's not depicted as frequently in many forms of media in the same way romantic breakups are, many other people have agreed and felt like it was a subject that needed more exploration. One of the things that made it so hard for me to understand relationship anarchy – a concept I'll explain more in depth later – was that I couldn't understand the concept of simply placing a value on relationships based on society's definition of them.

I suspect that you probably don't either. More likely than not, if your partner asked you to choose between them and your best friend, that probably wouldn't be a good sign. When you think of the way your heart works, you can only begin to really prioritize relationships when you're put in some type of dire situation that forces you to choose – which isn't the way we live our lives day to day.

The benefit you can find in challenging this assumption and trying non-monogamy is you will have more time to devote not just to dating others but also to friends and other relationships that should also be cherished, cultivated and valued.

Love is a scarce resource

Not only are we encouraged to believe romantic love is more important, but we're also encouraged to believe it's *scarce*. Narratives of 'soul mates' and 'true love' encourage us to believe that we can only really, fully and truly romantically love one person at a time. They encourage us to believe that the jealousy we may feel if our partner's eyes wander, especially for some men, is a sign of that love and passion that can only be truly felt for one person. What makes romantic love special, in our cultural narrative, is its rarity.

I don't believe this narrative has been pushed on us because it represents the way we really work as human beings or the way we should work. Growing up and being at odds with my own bisexuality, I was told frequently of how 'unnatural' gay relationships were. Despite the fact that you could point out countless examples of what could be classed as 'homosexual behaviour' in animals and in humans throughout history, many people were adamant that queerness was a new cultural phenomenon that didn't exist naturally or in the past. This led me to an exploration of our assumptions of 'normality'.

When I tell people in workshops about the existence of intersex people that blue used to be the 'girl colour' and pink used to be the 'boy colour', it baffles them because they have grown up with gendered expectations and roles as 'natural'. People who push the concept of gendered roles as natural are the same people who called queer people 'unnatural'.

Many assume gender roles are timeless and enduring. But both consumer capitalism and the media hold a powerful sway on our lives that we often forget and want to ignore. For example, many people today think rabbits eat carrots because Bugs Bunny eats them all the time – but Bugs Bunny's carrot eating is actually a cultural reference to Groucho Marx. Without that context, kids from my era just think rabbits love carrots when, in fact, they more often eat lettuce and greens.

There is a long history of the demonization of body hair on women that is intrinsically tied to body hair being racialized and hairlessness being seen as a sign of purity and cleanliness. Most babies wore long white dresses that made it easier to change them, bleach them and use them interchangeably between children, until the market wanted people to consume and created girl and boy colours to make it harder to use the same clothes for any new baby you had. Likewise, while I think monogamy is a choice that can work for many people, the fact that we're so encouraged to separate ourselves into two-parent family units that consume more than large co-operative communities is not merely a coincidence.

We are not really given any alternatives. We're given one trajectory in life that means success, which is monogamous marriage, and on top of that, if we're to secure the 'best' partner, we need to consume the correct diets, fads, clothing, accessories and whatever else in order to secure our 'mate'. Because love is scarce. And it requires a battle to retain and a battle to keep – both of which are fought primarily, and, again, this is no coincidence, by consuming.

When you pull back the curtain and see what we've been encouraged to believe about romantic love and love in general for what it is, you can then begin to understand and question whether every assumption you've made is true for you. You're probably capable of loving more than one person very deeply and easily. It's likely you've already done it, you've just, as many queer people have experienced with their romantic feelings, discouraged it, avoided it or chastised yourself for having those feelings.

Maybe this is the type of thing you only really begin to pick up on when you have a queer parent but...whenever someone tells you something is 'natural', always consider who profits from it the most.

The benefit you find in challenging this assumption and trying non-monogamy is less guilt and shame for feelings that might naturally occur to you and more freedom to explore them.

Sex and love are the same

This is an assumption that I feel like more and more people are challenging today so it might be something that's a little less on your mind. In fact, if you're anything like me and you're on the asexual spectrum you can feel like everyone else is 'hooking up', you aren't, and you don't understand the appeal.

However, what we practise when we're classed as 'single' isn't as easily transferable when we find ourselves in a partnership with someone else. Many people still see 'hooking up' as something you do until you properly 'settle down', meaning that you're not meant to be interested in having sex with others unless there's something fundamentally lacking in your monogamous relationship.

This is where the move to non-monogamy can be very tricky. For some people, monogamy does lack what they need to be happy in their lives, but that doesn't mean their partner isn't 'enough', though sexual differences and disparities may be what can drive someone into a situation where they feel like they must try non-monogamy. And when non-monogamy is happening because of a deficiency in a relationship, even if you don't feel that sex is love and love is sex, it can be incredibly difficult not to feel worried or jealous. Just because sex isn't love doesn't mean it doesn't have meaning or isn't important.

While some people may know sex and love aren't the same, they still believe that love should be prioritized over sex or that love can conquer any sexual incompatibilities within a relationship. In fact, the push to move to non-monogamy for the sake of helping a partner meet a sexual need that is not met through the relationship can come with a lot of resentment and very understandable feelings of inadequacy as much as they try to understand. Society has told them that their love should be enough.

Not only should we challenge the idea that sex and love are the same for the sake of asexual people who may want romantic love without sex, but also for the sake of the way intertwining these two can make us feel like our love for our partners should be able to supersede a sexual need. Sex and love are not the same...and love is not necessarily always more important than sex and sex is not necessarily always more important than love.

In my mind, the problem really isn't that love should conquer all these needs and it doesn't. It's more that we are encouraged to funnel all our needs exclusively through one romantic relationship when that may not be the reality of the way we want to do relationships – and considering the fact that elderly loneliness after losing a partner is such a huge issue, perhaps it's not the best way for any of us to prioritize relationships.

All relationships will end, whether through a 'breakup' or because one of the people within them dies. This isn't a comfortable thought for most people. While we've started to challenge taboos we've had around sexual needs and pleasure, there are still many taboos around death and dying that we've yet to challenge. The push to have one romantic partner who meets every single need ends up creating loneliness and sadness in our lives where there need not be.

The benefit you can find in challenging this assumption and trying polyamory could be that you're more sexually free to explore other options, but also that your circle of support isn't funnelled through a single individual (though I would also encourage monogamous people to expand their circle of support).

All relationships must take the same steps

Amy Gahran has invented an incredibly useful concept known as 'the relationship escalator' defined on her website 'Off the Relationship Escalator' and it's one of the things I refer to when I talk about the 'cultural script' of monogamy. We're encouraged through many, many avenues to see one path in life for our relationships and ourselves, and this has been true for a long time. While we no longer see romantic love as an impractical obstacle in securing a profitable 'match' for ourselves in terms of marriage, the idea of being monogamously married and usually with children is still very much embedded within our psyche as a sign of success.

Even if we are beginning to be more flexible in our understandings of when we should be married and that children are not always a choice people have to make to have a successful and fulfilling life, the concept of marriage or a 'commitment' gives us something that a lot of monogamous people take for granted that becomes difficult when people try polyamory. It's part of the cultural script that people follow that can reaffirm them in hidden ways. Because we have these steps of 'seriousness' into a relationship, they give us a sense of security, perhaps even a false one, that makes us feel like our relationship is less likely to break down.

The community and culture you're around also amplify the concept of relationship security. Many people highlight how difficult and awkward it can be when everyone among your friendship and peer group is 'settling down' and you aren't. In some cultures, the eyes on your back when you aren't following the cultural script your society has dictated to you can be an incredible pressure. It can be easy to take for granted how many people are available to help you with a relationship problem when you're monogamous and don't have to explain how differently your relationship works. Having the security of a culture that accepts and encourages you to partner monogamously, while a burden to many, still reinforces the idea of the security of monogamy taken in specific culturally defined steps.

The assumption that all relationships must take the same steps can feel suffocating and limiting to many people, even those who are monogamous. It can force people into situations and lifestyles that they don't really want because they feel like they have to in order not to 'miss out' on what society dictates is success. Many people end up finding non-monogamy much later in life after decades of monogamous marriage and, while they may love their partner, they would have chosen to do things differently if they had the option.

Some people are already challenging these concepts. Whoopi Goldberg, for example, has been called aspirational for her dislike of the concept of a traditional marriage and cohabitation (or, as she says, 'I don't want somebody in my house'). When they were together, Tim Burton and Helena Bonham Carter were known for their 'unconventional' decision to live in separate but adjoining houses in London, while doing so indicates a certain level of privilege. Even within monogamy, this cultural script of how we ought to live and do relationships doesn't have to dictate your life.

The benefit you can find in challenging this assumption and trying polyamory can be that you're more able to design relationships to fit your needs, although I would also encourage monogamous people to create a monogamy that fits their needs.

I wanted to avoid pointing out the obvious reasons you may think about when considering non-monogamy. Yes, you will get the chance to date and sleep with more people and that can be a huge benefit to many people for a variety of reasons. Some people are naturally flirtatious and love the process of dating and getting to know new people and polyamory offers them that opportunity.

For myself, I'm almost the exact opposite. I don't particularly enjoy people in general and I feel like whenever the planets align and I manage to find someone I like, I want the opportunity to see where that goes – that's my reasoning and benefit. I may wait longer to find a suitable partner or multiple partners, but it has usually been worth the wait and the hassle.

You may not have an immediate reasoning that springs to mind. You may not have an anchor right away and clinging onto the relationship you want to save may just be a temporary buoy you have until you can find an anchor – that's fine. Many people don't have everything figured out when they start having monogamous relationships and you shouldn't expect that either with non-monogamy.

What's most important is not approaching your exploration into polyamory with rose-tinted glasses. There can be a lot of benefits. I have pointed out previously in articles and here that there are a lot of social conventions tied into monogamy that aren't necessarily inherent to monogamy and breaking free of those can feel liberating, but that doesn't necessarily mean that polyamory or non-monogamy itself will be liberating for you personally or that you have to be non-monogamous to be liberated.

You need an anchor precisely because, in more cases than not, you will be weathering a storm. While some people may be able to take to polyamory and non-monogamy like a fish to water, others will struggle and not necessarily due to a personal failing. While I would encourage you to think of the benefits it can bring to your life, that doesn't mean avoiding the pain or fear that most likely will come.

CHALLENGE YOUR FEARS

Most people are afraid to lose the important relationships they have in their life. This is as understandable as it is inevitable. We must expect that our initial instinct when confronted with pain is to avoid it. I'm not particularly a fan of evolutionary psychology because I think it leads to a lot of assumptions about the concepts of nature and nurture, but I do think there is value in considering how our nervous systems have developed over time, the way that our societies and lives have changed so rapidly within the last hundreds of years, and how modern life impacts our nervous system.

It's less of the evopsych that people use to excuse misogyny and more what Robert Sapolsky talks about in *Why Zebras Don't Get Ulcers* about how our bodies respond to stress and how 'stress' used to be being chased by an apex predator and now it's receiving a difficult email – but our bodies react similarly. Clementine Morrigan writes brilliantly about being polyamorous and surviving trauma in her zine 'Love Without Emergency', especially about how attachment theory and PTSD can cause issues specific to people attempting polyamory. Though I don't really relate to attachment theory, I've found Clementine's writings about trauma and polyamory incredibly helpful in trying to unpack my fears and reactions.

When I was starting out in polyamory, I had the rose-tinted glasses I mentioned. The resources I had read told me not only that any fear I had of losing my partner was, without a doubt, jealousy but also that the best way to respond to jealousy was basically through a glorified self-pep talk. If convincing myself of my inner worth through positive self-talk worked, I would have solved my self-esteem problems long before I came across poly-amory. It seems like a good way to work through things because it isn't necessarily a bad approach overall, but if you couple the positive self-talk with a complete lack of acknowledgement of the validity of fears people feel and no desire to change some circumstances causing those fears, it's less assuring and more like self-gaslighting.

I'm sure taking a moment and recognizing the individual value you have to someone and recognizing that you have worth can work for a lot of people, especially those who have a momentary peak of anxiety but normally feel validated and justified. For those of us who have never had this reassurance in life, whose nervous systems are not always calm, who have recurring self-attack problems, or have faced constant bullying or trauma that makes their memories and first judgements of anything completely unreliable, this just isn't a suitable or viable solution.

Facing and challenging your fears isn't just a one-off process. It takes time and repetition. The most frustrating aspect of much beginner polyamory advice is the way it seems like dealing with any emotional difficulties that arise should be a one-off battle rather than a continuous effort, especially for those of us who have anxiety. Which isn't to say I'm eternally suffering under constant stress – but that it will and can rear its ugly head and not just occasionally. Learning how to cope with it in a way that makes sense and relies on something other than my ability to act as my own wingman is half the battle.

Accepting that anxiety is always a possibility

One of the reasons why the concept of giving myself a pep talk about how valuable I am worked so poorly for me was because it reinforced a harmful thought process that I actually needed to completely discard. This is something that I encourage all people to try when they're faced with an overwhelming fear and anxiety – especially as it relates to losing their partner.

Most of my anxiety within polyamory has come from the fear of losing my partner or partners for a variety of reasons. Sometimes my anxieties were founded in very logical conclusions drawn by my surroundings. Others and, to be honest, most of my anxieties were just there because I've been anxious pretty much all my life. My anxiety became more manageable when I stopped feeling like a failure and beating myself up just for having it.

The pep talk doesn't work when you have anxiety because anxiety is probably one of the cleverest and conniving thought processes you'll ever have the misfortune to come across. It will poke a hole in any theory you present and question anything that seems remotely airtight. For years, I tried to logic my way out of my anxiety and to beat it at its own game. My anxiety always transformed and adapted. The problem with the pep talk is, like any other way of rationalizing out of your anxiety, it may temporarily beat the anxiety back, but like cutting off the single head of a hydra, two will grow in its place.

So, if I told myself I had something unique to offer my partner, it would argue back that so does the other person they are seeing and whatever unique offering they had would outclass mine. The pep talks only made me wonder how unique I was and what *more* I could offer my partner to entice them to stay around. It was completely the wrong solution for me, and it backfired on me constantly.

Willing away my anxiety didn't work. And trying to outsmart it only gave it more ammunition against me. The first and clearest step in facing and challenging my fears was to admit I had them and that I wasn't a horrible person for having them. Most polyamorous people talk about relationship problems as if they maybe had them once, but no more. So, me admitting that I had problems and not having any shame for that was a huge step.

Identifying what you can control

Once you accept that anxiety is a part of your life, you're already doing the next step in some ways: identifying what you can control. Anxiety can come from a lot of different things depending on your background. For me, my anxiety and obsessive compulsions came from being in traumatic situations that were completely out of my control when I was younger. It's almost as if, since I could not fight the big monsters, my brain gave me little monsters and side quests to distract me in ways that temporarily made me feel like I had power and control.

When introduced to polyamory and to the thought process that I had unique features that would draw my partners in and essentially keep them around, it was a perfect storm. As a child coping with neglect, it was easier and better for me to believe at the time that if I was a perfect child, if I did everything right, then I could fix my surroundings and gain the love and attention I desired. Perhaps for people from more settled backgrounds, the suggestion that you have something unique to bring to a relationship is harmless, but for me it reinforced the worst of my anxiety.

It perpetuated the idea that I could control whether or not people loved or valued me through my actions or what I had 'to offer'. But the truth is, whether this self-pep talk is useful for you or not, no one, regardless of their background or self-esteem, has that type of control. And recognizing that and letting go, while it seems terrifying and agonizing, was what I needed to do.

Ultimately, you have to release the responsibility from your shoulders to keep your partner through your uniqueness. Now, you can always decide to be mean and hateful to your partner or never shower and *that* is something you can control, but outside of treating your partners and yourself as well as you can, there is only so much you can control. And that includes:

- whether or not your partner stays in love with you

- whether or not your partner stays attracted to you

- whether or not you and your partner are completely compatible

- whether or not you attract others

- whether or not you are attracted to others.

Point blank, if we could simply control whom, when, why and how we were in love with or attracted to anyone, the world would be much simpler. There are obviously things we can change, such as going out more to meet people or working on being more communicative, that can make us better partners overall. We can challenge our assumptions in a lot of ways and work on ourselves. But through your actions you can only control *who you become*, not whether or not someone appreciates or loves who you are. You have to let go of the ideal of perfectionism, which can be hard for people who grew up telling themselves that they could earn love by being perfect.

Removing the responsibility

If you've grown up in a traumatic environment or have had to deal with trauma, in that moment where you cannot change what's happening, it makes sense for your brain to tell you that if you do something differently, you can avoid the pain of the situation that you're going through in the future. In the moment, this is a coping mechanism that can keep you alive, empowered and away from plummeting into self-destruction.

Once you are not in that environment, this thought no longer serves you well for two reasons. The first is that, because so much is out of your control, it's unreasonable to expect yourself to be able to control everything that happens around you and the vigilance required for you to do so verges on paranoia.

The second reason is that you cannot believe this without also blaming yourself for what has already happened to you and putting the responsibility for preventing anything else directly onto your shoulders in a way that leads to more self-attack and self-blame. If you could prevent bad stuff from happening to you then you could have prevented what has already happened to you. Because so much is out of your control, putting all the responsibility to prevent something from happening to you completely on your shoulders is unrealistic.

Part of responding to some of your fears and anxieties is going to be evaluating how much is in your control and challenging whether you can actually, with your actions alone, control the outcome of what you're worried about. As easy as that sounds, this is quite difficult if you have believed for so long that you can control the outcome of events with your actions and that has soothed you for so long. It takes practice and effort and, most importantly, the next step.

Sitting with discomfort

Sometimes, recognizing and relieving yourself of the responsibility to manage and keep an eye out for all of the bad things that could potentially happen in your relationship and to you can be a huge relief, and that in and of itself may help eliminate a good deal of anxiety. However, recognizing something logically is miles away from knowing it in your bones.

Starting out in polyamory or in a new relationship is a risk. Even if your relationship is already well established, you are going off the beaten path. A lot of what makes the cultural script of monogamy so enticing for people to return to when they try polyamory is that society reinforces monogamy in a way that calms a lot of anxieties. And most of the time when people come to non-monogamy as an option, they don't remember the details of their first forays into monogamous relationships. They could have been just as nervous in their first monogamous relationship as they are now, but the memory doesn't feel as emotionally intense or as risky.

You're going to feel a certain amount of anxiety when building trust with a partner. Constantly in both my column and podcast I tell people that the first night, the first date or the first time your partner actually is with or could be with someone else can be really difficult. I'm not saying it definitely will be for you, but it can be fraught with anxiety. A lot of people advise first-time people to make adjacent plans the same night to distract themselves, but this may not be a possibility.

I have always found that the more trust I've built with a partner, the less and less anxiety I had, until I'm now excited to have a house to myself or a bed to myself for a period of time unless I've experienced something that's impacted my mental health. If you're brought to polyamory or non-monogamy because a partner is asking for it and you're struggling to find a good reason to try it yourself, the first night can be even more difficult without an anchor.

No one is going to be able to tell you if you can or can't do polyamory or if it's something that you want. Only you are going to be able to decide that. But I don't think that, if you experience a large amount of anxiety when the wheel finally hits the ground, that this means polyamory isn't for you. I wouldn't give everything up just because you're struggling at the start.

We will be looking in later chapters at active ways to support yourself and others during times of anxiety, but once you are able to challenge some of these thoughts, you're going to be able to avoid making rules out of fear and be in a better place to focus on your anchor.

ACTUALIZING YOUR NEEDS

Removing the responsibility from my shoulders to prevent bad things from happening to me and extending that to my understanding of relationships was one part of stepping towards a healthier understanding of how to have relationships, not only with others but also with myself. The next part was recognizing the power that I did have and what I actually could control.

I think too often people who have gone through trauma have experienced so much helplessness, especially if they were children when they went through the trauma, that they forget when they are an adult that they are not the same helpless child they once were. Once you stop blaming yourself for everything that has happened to you, you can actually shift too far into the opposite end of that – which is continuously blaming other people or other circumstances for things you have the power to change.

A good part of owning your needs and being able to not only ask for them but actually enforce boundaries that you put down will be trusting in and stepping into your own power.

Self-compassion

Forgiving myself and having compassion for myself for making the mistakes that I did led me to a place where I had a lot more compassion and forgiveness for others. I expected when I began therapy that I would turn into what I refer to often as an emotional gladiator, in that I would be less likely to experience such strong emotions. Instead, I ended up finding that I was already shutting myself off in a way that was not helping me connect to mine or others' humanity.

Before I started therapy, I used to watch a lot of horror films. While I still enjoy horror films now, I am definitely more emotionally affected by the distress of the people involved in them. I had always assumed that the triggers I had around sexual abuse scenes in films made me weak and that therapy would mean I could watch these unfazed. While I am less emotionally reactive to things in media that bother me, I am far more compassionate about all human suffering than I have been before.

Roxane Gay wrote an article in July 2021 titled 'Why people are so awful online' in the *New York Times* that reflected a lot of what I felt is true about online interactions – the capacity for anonymity and our collective sense of the lack of justice in the world creates a perfect storm. Furthermore, I think that even in person, not just within polyamory communities but in many others too, the ability to have power over others' reputations causes us to enact justice in unjust ways. I used to be supportive of this until I learned to have compassion for myself.

How people behave towards others is often partially a reflection of how they see themselves. If you cannot forgive yourself for previous mistakes, I believe you will find the road of trying non-monogamy to be even more difficult. My harshness with myself and my perfectionistic expectations of myself caused a good deal of my own problems. As early as possible, begin cultivating a relationship with yourself that is steeped in happiness and love rather than resentment and frustration.

Understanding your nervous system

After I learned that my anxiety was part of what was trying to keep me alive and sane, I also learned more about nervous systems. We really take for granted the way our modern lives are incredibly different from the way we've evolved over time. If you had told me that when my nervous system was agitated, I would be less likely to be able to learn or comprehend anything, I would have told you that that was ridiculous. I truly believed in the power of my own internal logical capabilities.

But the binary of logical/illogical when dissecting behaviours is something I've not found extremely helpful. Understanding my nervous system meant that I could actually make logical sense out of behaviours that didn't make sense to me and frustrated me. Instead of trying to see myself as belligerent or stupid, I began to understand why I had the feelings I had and what it was that I was trying to protect. But it also helped me understand others and their reactions as well and respect the need for space and centring myself before discussions or conflicts.

Most people are aware of the basic nervous system functions like fight or flight, but fewer know about two additional reactions: freeze or fawn. The complexities of these positions might be difficult for me to convey, given that I'm not an expert in these areas, but for me the biggest breakthrough was realizing that for some people a 'calm' nervous system is unnatural to them and they might seek out or attempt to do things that cause nervous system reactions because they feel so uncomfortable in the 'calm'.

I was able to see myself in that reflection. Not only was my anxiety a response to trying to help me feel empowered by creating imaginary situations I could 'control' through compulsion, but I was so unfamiliar with the state of a calm nervous system that my anxiety would often be triggered by it. I had to learn not only how my anxiety would work, but that it might also spiral not 'at random' but when I felt calmer. Quite often to my therapist I have described anxiety like rolling down a hill and collecting snow until you become a snowball. It felt uncontrollable and unstoppable, because I was focusing on trying to roll without collecting snow instead of stopping myself from rolling altogether.

I feel like understanding the nervous system is helpful especially for people who feel particularly removed from their emotions or have the experience of feeling compromised by emotions. When you understand that you can experience strong emotions without having a dysregulated nervous system, it changes your relationship to big emotions and makes them far less terrifying to face.

Self-control and responsibility

True crime is one of my special interests, which as an autistic person means it's something I could devote hours and hours of time to without getting bored. And I did. I remember I got to a point where every day at work I was listening to a true crime podcast and, when I wasn't listening to that, I was listening to Audible books about true crime. For hours and hours per day I marinated in some of the worst things that humanity has ever done to one another. After a while, I began to feel depressed.

It took me some time to figure out that it was the constant stream of negativity, despair and horror I was subjecting myself to that was causing my own depression, which caused me to be irritable and unhappy. I decided to stop listening to true crime podcasts, put a pause on watching any true crime documentaries or even horror films, and not read any more books about true crime or murder mysteries. I began to feel better almost immediately. Although true crime is still very much a big interest of mine, I now know I have a responsibility to myself to be a better guardian of my own mind.

In the past, I've talked a lot about the emotional responsibility we have towards partners while forgetting to emphasize the emotional responsibility we have to ourselves. It's likely because of something I'll explore in later chapters: that emotional responsibility can be used as a deflection technique. But it is also important for us to understand what responsibilities we have to ourselves. Unfortunately, it is not difficult to surround yourself with things that depress you or encourage you to feel helpless. I have seen that some communities can encourage a sense of personal helplessness and a lack of emotional responsibility. In many places, any impact you cause overrides the intent you have. Many communities encourage people to abandon all responsibility for their own emotions and always place the full blame on others any time we have a negative experience. While some people may have nefarious intentions, I believe that we're too often encouraged to give up our own agency in many spaces and to see ourselves as constantly victimized. A good deal of my therapy and healing has been about reclaiming my agency from both the experiences I have been through and the way I have constantly released that agency to others.

Because of my history with sexual abuse, I have always struggled with its depiction in media, especially when I have felt it's being done gratuitously. There have been times when I have felt so emotionally frustrated and upset with the lack of care and compassion I received when talking about sexual abuse to people who claimed to care for me, that I had no space for any understanding or differing perspectives on sexual abuse in media. I created a binary that felt safe to me: either you were with me, and you supported survivors and you wanted sexual abuse out of media, or you were a person who fetishized rape or worse, a rapist in waiting.

While I cannot control what I'm triggered by, to project that onto others and insist that others must have the same feelings as I do was me not taking responsibility for my own emotions and demanding others be identical to me so that I could be safe. I believe that a lot of survivors have this experience because we have felt so helpless in the past and continue to feel so in the future, even when our circumstances have changed. And while I think a warning system would still be helpful for me to have in films and TV shows, I no longer make such vast assumptions about the people who enjoy or create those types of media on such a grand scale.

Living under anxiety's thumb can feel disempowering and once we've removed the assumption that we can control everything, there is not much else to pull yourself back up with. But it's important to remember that we're not as hopeless as we once were. I made a choice when I decided to stop listening to so many true crime podcasts instead of continuing to choose to allow myself to slip further and further into depression. Given how interconnected the media is and how negative engagement means ad revenue for media sources, there is ample opportunity for us to bury ourselves in the negative, to focus only on the worst and to make ourselves miserable.

While we don't have control over a lot, we do have self-control, which we sometimes can forget to employ when we're so used to being controlled by anxiety. It's important to make active decisions in your life that contribute towards your overall mental health and wellbeing as much as possible. If this means limiting your access to certain people, places or things, it's definitely worth doing. Many of the problems I see in the podcast and column are situations where people may *feel* trapped, but they do have the power to pull themselves out. Always take responsibility for what you can control.

I realize that this philosophy can sound dangerously close to what a lot of survivors have been told in response to requests for empathy or even mentioning what they've been through. If you've been told to get over it, that it's not that bad, that you're wallowing in victimhood, that you're a martyr, that you've no reason to be so upset, there is an absolute unwillingness to see yourself as what you've always been told is shameful: being a victim.

I remember distinctly feeling so angry I was nearly shaking as I walked to the Student Life office at university to register myself as disabled. I was insulted and appalled by the very idea that I was not capable and saw the categorization of myself as 'disabled' as a mark of shame and felt an extreme amount of resentment for the narrative of myself as falling behind the growth and development of my peers. It took me a long time to understand that being disabled wasn't about wallowing in anything. Accepting certain things about my body and neurology as differences was actually part of taking responsibility for myself.

Likewise, recognizing what you can control and how your learned helplessness can contribute to your situation isn't about shaming yourself or about believing you can outperform any obstacle that comes your way. It's simply about recognizing not only what is out of your control, but also what is in your control and how you can change it. And it is far more empowering than believing you can do anything if you just put your mind to it. Remember that you are more powerful than you give yourself credit for.

Defining fulfilment

One of the things I frequently remind people is that polyamory is not about finding multiple unfulfilling relationships until you reach a level of permissible stasis. I think that a lot of people use polyamory to avoid a breakup so they can keep a relationship that is not serving them and get their essential needs met elsewhere. It's easy to be under the impression that your drive to find other partners is motivated by a desire to try to be polyamorous instead of a dissatisfaction with your current relationship.

A lot of people want to try polyamory to address a mismatch in a relationship's desires or wants. For example, if one partner identifies as asexual, a couple may open so that the other individual may be able to get their sexual needs met elsewhere. Depending on how you feel emotionally about being unable to provide something for your partner, this could be a relief or a constant reminder that you have 'failed' to provide something to your partner.

An incompatibility doesn't always have to mean a complete breakup and challenging the assumption that one partner must meet every single one of our needs can mean that we can accept that there is a difference in what we want out of relationships without that bringing the relationship itself to a crashing end. But one thing that I would encourage people to think about is whether, outside of a few basic incompatibilities, the relationship is actually *fulfilling*.

If you are in a place where your nervous system is constantly agitated, where you are fighting with yourself, where you are unhappy with yourself and where you are barely listening to yourself, it's going to be a struggle to really be able to see if a relationship is actually fulfilling. And if you're in need of just one person in your life who thoroughly understands you and you lack the support of a family circle, then it may feel like just having someone who cares about you is fulfilling in a way you can't live without.

I think it's important for people, monogamous or polyamorous, to be comfortable with not having any romantic relationships in their life, because if you're terrified of being single, you can end up staying in any kind of unfulfilling relationship simply to avoid being alone. Trusting that you can take care of yourself outside of a relationship, that you can have a fulfilling life without a relationship, is a really important step towards not just overall happiness but being able to figure out if a relationship is actually fulfilling to you.

While your ideal polyamory setup is typically about the logistics that work for you in your life, consider what those logistics say about your emotional wellbeing and personal fulfilment. There are larger questions about what you want out of life that you may not have had to consider because you've been given a narrative of general success to follow. But you have the capacity to define what fulfilment means to you and you alone and there's no time like the present to decide.

IDEAL POLYAM SETUP

One of the first exercises I encourage people to do when they're starting off in any non-monogamous or polyamorous setup is think about their 'ideal', usually in terms of the physical realities of how they organize their life – though there will be more to consider in the future.

When we consider monogamy, we have often been encouraged to varying degrees to think of our ideal partner, of specific idealized futures and of marriage for years, sometimes before we're near the age of entering relationships. So, when it comes to applying that imagination to polyamory or non-monogamy, there is a lot of time to make up for.

Go through the list below and rate each situation as 'ideal', 'low compromise', 'medium compromise', 'high compromise', 'hard limit' and 'not applicable':

Overall lifestyles

- Relationship anarchy . . . .
- Solo polyamory . . . .
- Kitchen table polyamory . . . .
- Parallel polyamory . . . .
- Don't ask, don't tell . . . .
- Open relationship . . . .
- Polyfidelity . . . .
- Triad . . . .
- Quad . . . .
- Swinging . . . .

- Monogamish . . . .
- Monogamy. . . . .
- Partners are out to family about non-monogamy

  . . . .
- Partners are out to friends about non-monogamy

  . . . .
- Partners are out to co-workers about non-monogamy

  . . . .
- Partners are out to no one about non-monogamy

  . . . .
- Getting married to one partner. . . . .
- Getting 'married' to multiple partners . . . .
- Having commitment ceremonies . . . .
- Eloping . . . .

Living arrangements

- Living with one partner. . . . .
- Living with two partners . . . .
- Living with three or more partners . . . .
- Living alone . . . .
- Living with roommates. . . . .
- Living with metamours. . . . .
- Living with family . . . .
- Living with children . . . .
- Living communally . . . .

- Sharing a bed . . . .
- Sharing a room . . . .
- Sharing a house . . . .
- Sharing transportation. . . . .
- Sharing house responsibilities . . . .
- Separate house responsibilities . . . .
- Temporary or part-time sharing or living

  . . . .
- Purchasing property together . . . .

Commonalities

- Sharing most hobbies. . . . .
- Sharing a few hobbies . . . .
- Sharing no hobbies . . . .
- Sharing the same friend groups . . . .
- Going on trips together . . . .
- Exercising together . . . .

Job/career

- Interacting with partner's colleagues. . . . .
- Attending work functions . . . .
- Working in the same company . . . .
- Working in the same department . . . .
- Working for the same boss . . . .
- Joining the same union . . . .

Children

- No children . . . .
- Birthing children . . . .
- Working with a surrogate . . . .
- Providing DNA for others' children . . . .
- Providing child support . . . .
- Adopting children . . . .
- Adopting stepchildren . . . .
- Fostering children . . . .
- Taking parental leave . . . .
- Being a godparent . . . .
- Having/adopting/fostering children before 35

  . . . .
- Having/adopting/fostering children after 35

  . . . .
- Providing primary childcare . . . .
- Providing some childcare . . . .
- Providing no childcare . . . .

Families

- Meeting direct family members (mother, father, siblings, etc.)

  . . . .
- Meeting extended family members (cousins, aunts, uncles, etc.)

  . . . .
- Attending family functions . . . .

- Hosting family functions. . . . .
- Sole partner introduced to family . . . .

Metamours

- Meeting metamours . . . .
- Befriending metamours . . . .
- Sharing trips with metamours . . . .
- Hanging out with partners and metamours. . . . .
- Dating metamours. . . . .

Political alignments

- Very aligning beliefs. . . . .
- Selective aligning beliefs. . . . .
- No alignment beliefs . . . .

Religious alignments

- Sharing the same religious affiliation. . . . .
- Sharing different religious affiliations . . . .
- Attending religious functions. . . . .
- Living with religious functions in the house

  . . . .

Money

- Pooling all money . . . .
- Sharing a single bank account . . . .
- Separate money . . . .
- Getting a loan together . . . .

- Saving together regularly . . . .
- Saving co-operatively with others . . . .
- Saving together for a specific goal . . . .

Use the space below to add your own lifestyle approaches.

. . . .

. . . .

. . . .

WORST FEARS

For many people who struggle with anxiety, this might be a difficult activity or something you already do ineffectively on a regular basis, but framing the activity this way might help ground you in trying to work out what you can and can't control.

For each section, outline what you feel one of your worst fears is regarding a specific relationship or relationships in general. You can choose to do this activity alone or with partners. It might be helpful at times to explore with your partners what your worst fears are so that you can get reassurance. Try not to get caught up in imagining the details of your worst fears unless you feel you need particular reassurance for that detail.

Once you outline them, try to create a risk percentage of how likely this is to happen. You can decide to do this based purely on your feelings or on a statistical risk of it actually happening – or both! This is designed to pull you a little back towards reality if you have a fear that is unlikely. Not all fears are necessarily unlikely.

After you've decided the percentage, decide what your mitigating factors will be to manage the risk or fear you have. Are there ways to prevent your fear from happening? Or ways to decrease the risk level? Think of things that both yourself and partners can do to accomplish this?

Once you've done that, think of your Plan B. During an event I attended in London, an artist named Speech Debelle said that when we're anxious, we're not actually anxious about the thing that we're fretting over, but we're actually afraid we won't be able to cope with what we're fretting over. Building confidence in your ability to cope with your worst fears will help. So, what's your Plan B? What will you do if this does happen? Whom will you reach out to for help? What actions can you take now to build your emotional resilience?

My worst fear:

. . . .
. . . .
. . . .

Risk percentage:

. . . .
. . . .
. . . .

Mitigating factors:

. . . .
. . . .
. . . .

My Plan B:

. . . .
. . . .
. . . .

SELF CHECK-IN

Having the time to reflect on your own decisions and circumstances may be something you do with a therapist if that is something you have access to, but it's also a practice you can cultivate with yourself through repetition. Take time, however frequently you need it, to check in with yourself and make sure you're heading down the path you want to be on instead of just following someone else.

Overall, do you feel like your life is heading in a place you feel confident with?

. . . .

. . . .

. . . .

. . . .

In what ways do you feel like you are being blocked from what you want?

. . . .

. . . .

. . . .

. . . .

What feels out of control for you at the moment?

. . . .

. . . .

. . . .

. . . .

Re-read your previous answer. Are there areas where you could take an active responsibility in changing this narrative?

. . . .

. . . .

. . . .

. . . .

What small steps will you take over the coming time period to change what feels out of control?

. . . .

. . . .

. . . .

. . . .

What changes do you want to see the next time you check in with yourself?

. . . .

. . . .

. . . .

. . . .

What do you think you will do if you do not see any changes?

. . . .

. . . .

. . . .

. . . .

What Will You Hear or Read?

∞

Once you start dipping your toes into communities or getting involved in some online forums, there are a certain amount of community-based issues you may come across. I have always described polyamory communities as a 'postcode lottery', which means that basically how good the community is really depends on where you are. I have heard of incredibly toxic communities and incredibly affirming ones. I've been in 'the community' and also have had communities with people who are just as polyamorous but don't get involved in polyamory-themed events or consider themselves a 'polyamorous community'.

Still, there are a lot of common factors you may end up coming across when you start to read your first bunch of books or go to events. I experienced a lot of these when I began first getting involved in the community near me so I'm hoping pointing some of these out might help you take on your community with a little bit more information behind you than I had.

JEALOUSY

I have, in the past, described jealousy as polyamory's Scarlet Letter. It's the first question most monogamous people ask when you say you're polyamorous – 'Don't you get jealous?' – and it's associated and tied up with so many negative things in the polyamory community that almost no one will admit to feeling jealousy and, if they did, it was just once and they gave it up a long time ago.

What is jealousy?

I have a bone of contention with the definition of jealousy or the way most people seem to define it. In my own experience, I have made the mistake of assuming any negative feeling I had was jealousy and that jealousy was always a bad, negative thing that I had to purge myself of. Sometimes I still have moments of panic where I wonder if I'm jealous, but most of this comes from the shame that I picked up from the polyam literature I read first.

I find it more helpful to define jealousy as, specifically, wanting something that your partner has or wanting something they are giving to someone else. Personally, the moment of my life when I felt jealous, and I was absolutely sure I felt it, was before I had my breast reduction. I witnessed other trans people get surgeries they needed because they had a family who could pay for them, or they got their surgeries approved on the NHS. Without a doubt, that felt like intense jealousy. This was nothing like what I was feeling when I thought I was being 'jealous'.

More importantly, I don't feel like being afraid of losing your partner or your relationship should be defined as 'jealousy', especially since the types of approaches I would recommend when someone is afraid of losing their partner are not the approach I would advise if your partner has something that you want for yourself (either literally, in the form of a getting a date with someone who rejected you, or figuratively, like financial stability).

Regardless of how you personally define jealousy, the approach that is often advised for people to attempt, in my experience, is yet another self-pep talk that doesn't help or even makes the problem worse. And the shame that surrounds jealousy almost always characterizes it as a feeling that is without merit or is solely rooted in self-hatred, with self-hatred being conflated with insecurity. Jealousy isn't always just about self-hatred or insecurity, or even without merit.

What is insecurity?

One of the biggest conflations in a lot of polyamory advice is the assumption that jealousy, in whichever way you define it, comes from 'insecurity'. But when a lot of people say 'insecurity', what they generally mean is self-hatred. Allow me to split a few more hairs here.

Insecurity is when you don't feel secure, to put it plainly. Without a doubt, having self-hatred can cause you to feel insecure, but it's hardly the only thing that does. When we're starting out in polyamory, we're trying something, as I've mentioned, with no cultural script and no societal confirmation of 'success'. In many cases, some people trying polyamory are doing so to keep a relationship that they fear they may lose, not because they actually want to try it.

People who have loads of self-confidence and don't hate themselves can still feel insecure in new and uncertain circumstances. If we consider what are defined roughly as the major stressors in life (e.g. moving, having a child, job loss, death of a loved one, etc.), regardless of whether the overall situation is good, I believe that opening your relationship is a major life stressor.

I doubt seriously we would suggest that a person who is feeling afraid, sad, nervous or scared after having a new child or moving to a new town is only feeling that way because of their personal 'insecurity' so why do so many always assume that someone who is feeling jealous, regardless of how you define it, is only feeling so because of a personal fault?

What people generally mean is that if you feel you have no internal value and if you hate yourself you are more likely not to believe you have any value to a partner and you're then more likely to be jealous and afraid of your partner spending time with others. Many people think of 'jealousy' in the toxic monogamy sense where a guy, usually, is enraged by the very thought of their partner even looking at another man. As a result, we stereotype the very feeling of jealousy itself with controlling behaviour and assume they go hand and hand with self-hatred and insecurity.

But you can be insecure in a new relationship style because you're afraid to lose your partner without hating yourself, thinking you're worthless, or feeling the need to react with explosive anger or attempt to control them. The problem can sometimes come when we're in relationships that don't meet our needs, ignore that our needs aren't being met, and then we end up feeling self-hatred because we assume *we* must be the problem.

Conflating jealousy with controlling behaviour and insecurity with self-hatred doesn't help people address either the problems they are personally having or the problems that may be happening within a relationship. It encourages people to believe 'jealousy' is only a personal problem that you must handle yourself and ignores the fact that jealousy could be an understandable feeling that comes from an unmet need.

Wanting something your partner has

Let me first address the solution to what I think is actual jealousy – wanting something that your partner has.

The solution for this *isn't* to give yourself a well-earned self-pep talk but to think about the reasons why you want what your partner has. These can sometimes be unavoidable things that your partner can't do anything about and going to them for reassurance about it might not be that helpful.

So many times, in the podcast and in the column, I've seen people afraid to date or commit to other people until their partner is also committed to or dating someone else to keep it 'fair'. It seems almost normal for couples just opening up to experience one person having a lot more 'luck' when it comes to dating than the other – and I put the luck in quotes because I think too often people mistake a lot of interest in dating you as success when it can actually be overwhelming or that 'interest' can actually be sexual harassment.

Even if what you're feeling is jealousy, it might be extremely valid. If one partner has a lot more skill in speaking to people and is more confident, they might be able to get more dates. Being jealous of that doesn't make you a bad person nor does it mean that you're immediately going to jump towards controlling your partner. If we can acknowledge that we live in an unjust world that privileges certain people over others and that some people may still have some work to do on themselves towards being more confident and happier, then we can also understand that these power dynamics don't magically disappear when we log in to dating apps.

And dare I say it, even if we were to take someone like the stereotypical jealous boyfriend whose behaviour borders on or crosses the boundaries of abusive, when we deconstruct those behaviours they may also come from a fear that is relatable to most, though this doesn't excuse abusive behaviours. Jealousy is an emotion that most of us will experience regardless of how confident we think we are. The emotion itself is not 'toxic' or bad. What matters is what we do with the emotion.

And I would further argue that it isn't just jealousy that creates situations where people are controlling or attempting to control their partner, it is also *entitlement*. People can feel entitled without feeling jealous at all. One of the most common things that people who abuse or hurt others have – whether their behaviour stems from past trauma, brain structure, inadequate socialization or anything else – is the assumption of entitlement.

It can be difficult when we struggle with mental health and, especially if we have dealt with abuse in our lives, to claim our right to basic needs without feeling 'too much'. Being around people who felt entitled to our space and our lives can make us feel like we don't even have the right to breathe. Working out whether you're coming from a place of entitlement or a place of having a need is something you should work on with a therapist. It's possible that it could be both.

Learning how to self-advocate is something that will take confidence to build and learn and we can all, as flawed humans, have moments of entitlement where our privilege gets the best of us. Part of coping with this has to do with relieving yourself of the responsibility to always be right and be perfect, which can cause as much anxiety as always expecting yourself to fail. Mistakes will always be made. Being a person willing to apologize and also being around people who do not put you on a pedestal is critical.

When it comes to this type of jealousy, working on your own to figure out how you can get your needs met rather than trying to get reassurance from your partner is probably the best bet. There may be some material ways your partner can help, but if there aren't then it might not be helpful for them to give reassurance about this. For example, a straight partner could not make queer dating any easier for me and, unless we discussed it and they could cope with me whinging about it to them when I'm jealous they have a date, I would probably find another community to talk about it in.

Wanting something your partner gives

This is similar to the previous section, but I separated it since the answer to this goes a little bit deeper. One of the biggest experiences I have had with jealousy was in a relationship where my partner and I lived together and I was incredibly lonely. I assumed that wanting another partner made me *super actually* polyamorous but, really, I wanted another partner because the partner I had wasn't devoting the time or attention to me that I needed.

For me, one of my needs in relationships, even friendships, is quality time. If I feel like a burden to someone or if they don't really pay any attention to me or if I feel they think being around me is a chore that they don't want to do, then that absolutely kills the relationship for me. At the time, I assumed that I was lucky to have a partnership where someone wasn't physically or verbally abusive, so I didn't realize things weren't working for me.

I assumed that any negative feelings I had about the relationship were a result of my insecurity – and that seemed incredibly likely since I *was* very insecure about a lot of things. I had anxiety and constantly questioned my own perceptions of everything and always assumed I was not only at fault but powerless to fix anything. If my partner wasn't interested in grocery shopping for me when I was tired, I took that as a sign that I was a burden and, therefore, it was my fault. After a while, the rejection became so painful that I just stopped asking and that seemed to temporarily solve the issue. I also tried to look inward and see value in myself, but that didn't result in me magically getting what I needed either, especially when I stopped asking for it.

When my partner got up early one day to buy fresh fish to make sushi for a friend who was visiting, I absolutely lost my shit. I was so upset about it that I stayed at a friend's house that night. Something so seemingly small that shouldn't be a big deal became a huge deal because of what it represented, and I was completely and utterly jealous. Not because I wanted my partner not to do anything for anyone else or because I didn't want them to date this person, but because I desperately wanted them to do something like that for me.

Sometimes you can become jealous because of an unmet need. If your partner promised to take you to a specific restaurant and kept making excuses and they took another partner there, you would probably feel jealous. Even if the unmet need is small, it tends to be about what's not happening in a relationship that you want to happen. These types of relationship problems can happen within monogamy – where one person wants something from their partner and isn't getting it. The difference is that when we witness our partners give something to other partners that they aren't giving to you, that can be especially painful. And when new relationship energy or NRE is hitting a partner really hard, it can be particularly difficult.

The best way to address this type of jealousy is directly. If there is something your partner is giving to other partners or doing for other partners that you want, you have to ask for it directly. Not every single incidence of this is necessarily malicious. Asking directly for an unmet need isn't easy at all and being rejected outright puts out larger questions about whether the relationship itself is serving you, which may be why we want to avoid asking outright. But the sooner you're able to recognize you're not getting what you need and learn to ask for it, the better.

But unfortunately, if you make the mistake I did, you can spend a long time ignoring it and believing it's a result of your own insecurity, especially thanks to the way jealousy is advised about in the community. Your partner's reassurance isn't going to change an unmet need. They have to actually meet your need or admit they do not want to; reassurance from yourself or your partner will only keep you floating; it won't get you out of the water.

Being afraid of losing your partner

Many people have told me that the above definitions of jealousy actually describe *envy* and being afraid of losing your partner *is* actually jealousy – or all of the above are jealousy. The reason I separate them is not to be annoying about how we define words, though I do think it's important, but because I think that being afraid of losing your partner is fundamentally different from the previous two issues.

Wanting something your partner is getting or giving to someone else is primarily about an unmet need within your relationship or your life overall. Sometimes that unmet need is a thing your partner can address and sometimes it isn't. But your relationship can be meeting all your needs and you can *still* be afraid to lose your partner. You can be confident and self-assured, and *still* be afraid to lose your partner.

In fact, I would argue that for people with anxiety and for people starting off in a new relationship, whether or not they've been polyamorous or non-monogamous for a while, it's pretty common to be afraid of losing your partner. I think that monogamous people also have those fears when they start a new relationship. Even when dating people fear that someone new may stop liking them or may change their mind. There are endless jokes about people being afraid their long-term and married partners don't actually like them and needing that to be reconfirmed.

For many people, this isn't a sign that there's something deeply wrong in and of itself, but it could actually be a fairly regular state of being for a while into a new relationship until you establish some trust and time with each other, especially if you lean towards feeling particularly anxious. I do think that being afraid of losing your partner, even if it's not what I would define as 'jealousy', can *still* lead to controlling behaviour. Often because both people in a couple who open up fear losing the relationship, they will do things like only looking for a closed triad or seeing another person as a 'third' so that they don't have to risk losing their relationship.

The best way to address being afraid is first and foremost to accept that you're afraid and that this is a typical reaction when you're opening up or trying polyamory for the first time. Reassurance from your partner in this case *can* help, but be wary about turning reassurance into a competition. Too many people reassure their partners when opening up with things that invite comparison and create hierarchies. Even if they mean the best when they tell their partner that 'You are the most important to me', when you create a pedestal, even if you are currently the one placed on it, it also means you can be kicked off.

Ultimately though, facing your fears will be part of addressing this, and realizing how little control you have over the situation can help counteract this. While you could be afraid of losing your partner because you do have self-hatred and believe that you have nothing to offer your partner, I doubt that just giving yourself a pep talk or recognizing the uniqueness of your 'offering' will help you. When you have self-hatred that runs that deep, it's complicated to address and requires more work, but that doesn't mean reassurance from your partner doesn't help along the way.

Ways to address jealousy

No matter how you define 'jealousy', thinking that the solution is always to focus inward, assuming that the responsibility is entirely on your shoulders to work out and blaming yourself isn't the best way to go. While other people may have felt differently, the advice that I read for people starting out in polyamory encouraged me to group any negative feeling I had in the 'jealousy' bin and assume it was my problem to handle.

In my first ever technical experience of polyamory, I ignored some of my feelings and assumed my discomfort was because I hadn't yet escaped the mental confines of monogamy. I compare this a lot to how I assumed my asexuality was me being a prude and tried to push past my discomfort anyway rather than accept my feelings or lack thereof. The experience ended with me finding out that he was using me to cheat on someone else. Had I not ignored my feelings for so long, I would have avoided a lot of hassle.

My worry with the way people advise others to cope with jealousy is that, rather than learning how to do positive self-talk and learning the concepts of regulating their own nervous system, people end up in a cycle of self-blame and self-attack. Advising people who have mental health problems or who come from abusive backgrounds where they were gaslit constantly to question their initial assumptions about their feelings can be a setup towards absolute failure.

Perhaps people who are more neurotypical benefit from the idea that they should question themselves, but people who struggle with mental health issues can struggle with the exact opposite – being so trapped in a constant questioning of your own feelings and thoughts that you seem incapable of connecting to what's real, let alone finding enough purchase to grasp a hold of and reassure yourself.

Finding a way through the maze of what you may feel and picking out what's coming from unmet needs, what's coming from a fear of losing your partner and what's coming from just you being anxious in general is fraught with difficulty and is nowhere near as simple as advice, even my own, can make it sound. But take one thing out of the equation – blaming and attacking yourself for feeling anything at all – and it might make the process just a little bit easier.

INDEPENDENCE

Polyamory as a practice isn't necessarily modern but the word 'polyamorous' and polyamorous communities are new things. Most of my experience within those communities has been in the United States and the United Kingdom and, in these communities, individualism is reinforced in a lot of advice and introductory information.

Despite personal independence being seen as an important value in many English-speaking and European countries, the type of monogamy that's encouraged socially tends to foster an unhealthy codependency. As I've mentioned previously, society encourages people to see their one romantic partner as the person who should meet all their needs and not to rely on friendships, family and other resources. Which isn't to say that people can't have families or friends, but there is often a lot of suspicion cast on monogamous people who are too close to friends or don't seek their partner to meet their immediate needs first.

As a result of this combination of contradictions, independence and individualism are highly valued in a lot of polyamory communities and writing. While I don't think independence is necessarily a bad thing, what's encouraged in polyamory advice can easily be taken by people who struggle with poor mental health, who are afraid of being considered a burden, who may already have been told by society that they are too 'needy' and morphed into something that encourages isolation and self-attack.

No human is an island

When I first heard of polyamory, I was interested in it mostly because of the co-parenting opportunities. A big aspect of the motivation for me to pursue polyamory was so that I could have as many children as possible and also the help that I needed because I've always felt like more parents can give a large family a lot more support.

The more I understood my disability and the way it might impact me as I aged, the more I also realized that I would need taking care of potentially in the future too, though this seemed at odds with the polyamory values of independence. The advice and introductory materials that I read encouraged me to avoid being 'controlling'. Along with jealousy, it seemed to be one of the worst things you could be.

While I don't think that those who wrote some of the introductory materials I read wanted me to think that I couldn't tell people about my problems, the assumption that one can always judge when one is asking too much of a partner is not really true for everyone. Having a disability only further compounds the issue because, especially knowing that I might eventually have to rely on others more, I felt even less like I wanted to involve other people in managing any of my feelings and wanted to handle everything myself.

This was before I had questioned much of the ableism I had internalized. I had always assumed that it was up to me to catch up to everyone else who was 'normal' and that the ways I needed to rely on anyone else were things I should avoid and feel shame over. I pushed myself into situations that I was uncomfortable in and didn't communicate how I felt because I assumed my feelings were ridiculous or wrong. Any time I needed reassurance or could have used it, I didn't seek it out because I assumed all the problems were my own to fix. While many events aren't great with accessibility, I quite often didn't give people the chance to meet those needs because I assumed they were too much to ask for.

One of the biggest turning points for me in understanding the balance I could strike between supporting myself and asking for help from others was learning more about the way disability is constructed by society. This isn't to say that it's society's fault I don't produce hormones, but whose needs are considered 'special' and whose needs are considered typical are defined by society. Understanding that my neurology wasn't less than, just different, helped me understand that I wasn't a worse or bad partner just because my needs might be different.

Throughout the column and the podcast, I remind people that there is a reason that solitary confinement is considered torture and why our brains cannot handle it. We're a social species that has survived through interdependence. A certain level of independence is helpful, especially if you're struggling to find people who can actually provide support to you in your immediate area, but it's important to avoid taking the independence that's offered in the material that you read so seriously that you begin to feel ashamed to ask for help.

Managing your emotions

Another frequent argument which encouraged me to avoid asking my partners for help or even holding people accountable for their actions was one I would hear echoed in many communities: no one is responsible for your emotions except you.

While I do think it's important to recognize that blaming other people for causing your emotions is reductive, disempowering and, at worst, manipulative, the idea that a person has no responsibility for the emotional pain they cause can be used just as harmfully. Polyamorous people can be just as cruel and intentionally harmful as monogamous people, even taunting their partners into tears. The idea that someone isn't responsible for that, even if their partners could have been 'stronger' to avoid being upset, doesn't sit right with me.

Emotions are a difficult thing to control and there have been times when I've felt I can't control my own emotions, especially if they are tied to a breakdown I'm having because of sensory overload. We clearly can't control exactly how we feel at all times. If we could, then emotions we didn't want to feel like grief or sadness would be far easier to cope with. However, even if we can't control our emotions, we can learn to manage and cope with them.

Not all of us are given the tools to manage our emotions adequately under pressure. Not all of us are able to adequately recognize and categorize our emotions quickly. Rather than saying, 'No one is responsible for your emotions except you', what might be more helpful is, 'You are responsible for the actions you take and their consequences, even if you did them under duress'. But we also have to clarify, in that statement, what we mean by responsibility.

We have to be responsible for the actions we take, even when we're under duress and our brains are in survival mode. Being responsible for those actions can mean apologizing if we feel we did something wrong and trying to make amends to the party we've affected, if possible, as well as working towards not making the same mistakes again. Part of extending an apology also has to be not expecting instant forgiveness or seeking absolution. Sometimes, when we have hurt people, whether intentionally or not, they do not want us to be in their lives. I don't believe apologies made from a place of shame are effective and I don't think it's an actual apology if people are apologizing because they feel they have no other choice; people who have done wrong also have to understand that the other person may need boundaries for their own protection.

Beyond the realms of right and wrongdoing, responsibility within a relationship involves showing up and honouring a commitment you make to each other. That's why it's so important to have a discussion about your expectations when you enter a relationship. This may explain the gap in experiences between single people who have loads of fun playing with couples and other single people who feel like they've been used and chucked by a couple when things got rough. Making expectations clear helps everyone involved.

I have an entire category of my column devoted to 'emotional responsibility and metamours' and most of them include a very common scenario I witness: a hinge who does not know how to adequately balance the emotional responsibility of two partners and, quite often, people who aren't the hinge who are trying to make peace with a metamour or make their partner's partner like them. I've witnessed many situations where a hinge doesn't want to take responsibility for setting their own boundaries, making decisions about how they spend their time or addressing situations head on, and instead avoids them or blames a partner for their unavailability. And more than a few situations of people dating so many people they don't have the time to actually be available in any real way to any of them.

While it's not necessarily a hinge's responsibility to play referee between two or more of their partners who don't get along as the others are adults who can set their own boundaries, if you decide to cancel a date with one person for another, you can't just blame that on the other person. If you know the commitments you've made to both people and you can communicate those clearly, you can usually work things out, but too many times I see people blaming a partner instead of taking that responsibility.

Some take 'independence' to mean that they do not have to be responsible for their choices and instead blame others for their actions. The concept that 'no one has responsibility for your emotions but you' can be helpful when someone puts the responsibility for all their happiness on your shoulders. Be wary, though, that others can use this phrase to absolve themselves (in their mind) of having to apologize to you for hurting your feelings. Generally, it's always wiser to focus on who is doing the action and whether or not they are actually willing to see that through.

Too much information

Some people attempt to solve their anxieties in polyamory by asking to know everything or even wanting or needing to be in the room any time that their partner is with someone else, usually sexually. People can make these types of arrangements for a variety of reasons. There are some people who are exhibitionists/voyeurs and who like being a part of or hearing about their partner's exploits. That isn't necessarily a harmful thing so long as the other person is aware and has consented to everyone being a part of, even in an indirect way, their sex lives.

I don't think that when people use this as an approach they are necessarily distrusting of their partners. It rarely ever comes from a place of believing that their partner will cheat on them and almost always comes from a place of being worried about unclarity or a breakup – even when both people agree to these types of terms. People seem to think unconsciously that knowing and witnessing what their partner is doing will somehow prevent something terrible from happening.

Sometimes this can be somewhat helpful because, if they are there to witness their partner being intimate with others, they can't really live in a state of denial or pretend their partner is monogamous with them. Wanting to directly expose yourself to the reality of the situation can in some ways help you cope with it in a better way than avoidance would. But I think that it also puts you through a lot of unnecessary and potentially painful things that you don't need to experience just to accept the full reality of non-monogamy.

There are lots of different ways to do polyamory. For some people, they want all their partners to get along and form a big family. Others would rather have a style where their relationships were very separated, and their partners rarely meet. It's easy to get trapped in the idea that, despite the fact that so many say there is no one right way to do polyamory, the 'best' way is clearly one where all of your partners get along and everyone is best friends. And it can be easy to feel like you're failing if that isn't the way you do things.

People also, understandably, as they do in monogamous relationships with their partner's family members, think that if their metamours do not like them, this could have some effect on their partner's feelings about their relationship. While they may not think that their metamour would issue a veto or expect their partner to dump them, the path of least resistance is one where you, as a new partner who may feel in competition with others who have been with your partner for longer, want to make things as smooth as possible. Especially if you've been in an abusive relationship at any point where you've been made to feel like you caused the behaviour of whoever hurt you, you can feel scared about causing your partner strife and about that strife getting in the way of your relationship.

You can't inoculate yourself against the pain of a breakup by exposing yourself to seeing and knowing exactly what your partner does with others. That just isn't how it works. And seeing what your partner does with others isn't necessarily going to make you more secure, more capable of handling things, or allow you to identify a problem before it becomes unmanageable. If you have agreed and discussed the issues of the privacy of the third party with your partner and they find it interesting or hot to hear about your dates or your life with your other partners, then great. But if not, you're putting yourself through a whole mess of hurt and discomfort that won't actually solve anything.

Some people are really worried about having a relationship where their partner gets to pretend that they are monogamous and feel it's dishonest to keep the details away from their partner. Whenever you're sharing or asking to hear details, it's always important to ask yourself equally why you want to know this information, or you want your partner to know, and what benefits it will bring. Compare the questions you ask about their other relationships with other areas of their life that are just as important. Really examine whether you feel you have something to prove and if not knowing that information brings you anxiety that you should perhaps be examining.

The limits of reassurance

It's ironic that there is a lot of focus on independence within many polyamory communities but also an insistence that reassurance from your partner can solve a lot of the problems that people have with polyamory starting out. While the point of this chapter is to discourage you from attempting to solve all the problems that you encounter on your own, it's also important to recognize what the limits of reassurance are.

Reassurance isn't the be all and end all, as clichéd as it may sound, actions do speak louder than words. A partner who *tells* you that you mean the world to them isn't the same as a partner who actually *shows* you that you mean something to them through decisive action. And if you read any book about abusive relationships, you know that after a period of abuse there is usually a period of apologetic remorse where a partner verbally and frequently promises not to hurt their partner again.

In some cases where your problem stems from the relationship not working for you because your partner either can't or isn't willing to meet your needs, reassurance may actually provide a temporary serotonin boost that makes you able to stay in the situation you're in for longer instead of actually seeing it for what it is. It's, as I've said before, like blowing air into a lifejacket with holes. It works only in the temporary and not in the long term.

As I've also mentioned in the previous section on jealousy, if the problem is not something your partner can actually change or do anything about, and especially if they are not experiencing the same issues, they may not be able to do much to comfort you. I think we see and recognize this when it comes to our friends. If we're going through, for example, a particularly difficult death such as that of a close family member, we might seek out friends who have had similar experiences. Not because we don't believe that our friends who haven't gone through this are unable to give us help, but because we want to hear from someone who can empathize with our situation.

Not to mention, a lot of people seek a level of reassurance from their partner that they're not really able to provide. To quote another cliché, they say money doesn't buy happiness for a reason: because close relationships with others just aren't things you can replace. Likewise, reassurance cannot stand in for building a positive relationship with yourself.

Whether you're monogamous or polyamorous, you still have to cultivate a relationship with yourself and prioritize your own needs so that you can actually show up fully for other people. Without a doubt, having both positive relationships and other stable nervous systems can help you stabilize your own and have a self-esteem boosting effect.

I think this is probably what people mean when they encourage independence because so much of mono-centric culture encourages people to see themselves as half of one whole and complete themselves through a monogamous relationship. And while I think it's wholly possible that some people thrive better in romance than they do alone, that doesn't mean ignoring your needs or feelings and becoming codependent. Your partner cannot cure or fix any of the integral issues you have with yourself.

I have certainly experienced partnerships that enabled me to have a better relationship with myself. Partners can provide a stable ground for you to take an emotional risk that you would not take alone. I know I have had partners who have helped me learn how to state my needs better and that has had a positive impact on me overall, but I still had to do the work.

The point isn't to say if you ever have a problem you shouldn't seek reassurance, but you should be aware of its limits. Don't ask your partners to be your therapist. Your partner can't be an objective third party in every situation and expecting reassurance to help you be happy with yourself or with a relationship might just end up dragging painful situations out for longer.

Know whom you can depend on

My retort to the concept of independence isn't that you should always rely on your partners and abandon yourself, but that you need a combination of independence and interdependence. We'll address this more in later chapters when we talk about self-care, partner care and community care, but suffice to say, it's just not as simple as trying to weather a storm alone. There can be real challenges when it comes to this because you might be like me and not have any family systems to rely on while your partner does. Or, you may have family, but they aren't people you can actually rely on.

If you've recently moved, you may have no immediate community in your area, or if you're practising polyamory in a conservative area, you may not only not have any community to discuss problems with, but you also might not even be able to discuss basic things with people like colleagues without fear of retribution. Therapy is an option for regaining some sense of support but it's not a realistic option for many people due to cost or availability. Talking to your metamours about a shared partner is sometimes complicated and not the best way to go about solving the problem so it becomes less of an option. Polyamory can sometimes be very isolating and independence may be your only option.

Perhaps the reason why the advice on how to handle some of the struggles that come with polyamory is hyper-focused on independence is because so much of it can be realistically out of our hands or control. We can only really focus on how much we support ourselves and offer our partners reassurance where we can. Still, it's important for us to realize the limits both individual independence and dependence on our partners have in terms of solving some of our problems. A lot of the first times you experience in polyamory will be anxious times for most and reassurance unfortunately can't prevent that.

PROBLEMS WITH COMMUNITIES

As I've said, polyamory communities can be 'postcode lotteries'. By that, I mean that the quality of the type of community that you'll find can vary widely depending on where you live and what's in your area. You may not even have enough people that can actually make a community. Very few communities, even large ones, have the funding available to be able to pay people to run community events.

A lot of communities have this issue and what it means for representation is that only the people who are available to commit a lot of time to something unpaid are able to hold power and visibility within communities.

What makes 'a community'?
It makes sense when you're starting out to want to find a group of people who know what they're doing. It's often the advice people have regarding issues around sexuality or other aspects of our personalities that might be marginalized or not understood by a lot of people. This also goes in line with what I've said previously about being a social species. We want to feel like we're not completely alone and many of us have varying levels of tolerance in terms of how we cope with loneliness.

We have the extraordinary benefit of being able to access the Internet, which also no doubt comes with its downsides. It does allow for us to find communities that can work for us, although sometimes it's also a struggle when you run into communities that don't work well for you. Building your own community online can often come with less difficulties and time constraints than building an in-person one, meaning that more people have access to this ability and it's not solely something that people with a variety of privileges can do.

A community at its simplest can be a group of people you share a common bond with, but I think that a useful and supportive community is made up of people, just like partners, who have a vested interest in your wellbeing. I think that when we're feeling alone and we're looking for other people who are in a similar situation to ours, we often *assume* they have a vested interest in our wellbeing, but unfortunately that isn't always the case. You can be actively involved in a community, do tons of work for that community, and even put your heart and soul into it, only to find out that community has no interest in your wellbeing – in the same way you can in a relationship.

Even if you have the ability to sacrifice your spare time for a community because you don't work more than 40 hours a week, don't have a disability that takes time to manage, don't have children (or you might have all these but still push through anyway), you can still end up being taken advantage of by a community in the same way a person can take advantage of you. What's important, just as with individual relationships, is to make sure that the community is reciprocal in terms of what it's offering you.

Community leaders

One of the things I've warned about in the column or podcast is not to assume that people who lead communities or seem to have a lot of people following them in general are somehow better at polyamory or safer. Unfortunately, we tend to assume that the more partners people have, the better they clearly are at relationships. I get the thought behind it because it logically seems like that would be the case. Especially if this person seems already 'vouched for' by the community. That must be why they're in charge of things, right?

While it may be a result of the postcode lottery in my area, my experience has been that a number (not all, but a good deal) of the people I encountered who were in charge of things or popular in the community have been some of the worst people in any community that I have ever met. Many people who go through anxiety daily feel somewhat more comfortable when someone they're around has confidence. Sort of like if you have social anxiety, it's easier to go to parties and other social events if you have a confident, outgoing person who will stick by your side the whole night.

Sometimes when you get caught in the beam of attention of someone who is popular and confident, it can feel like they are caring for you. Or, if you're like me and you've been through any amount of neglect growing up, positive attention can be addictive, and you can be drawn to it like a moth to a flame. Aspects of growing up can poke their heads out in a really ugly way in terms of thinking you have more value because someone who has more social capital is paying attention to you.

But as I mentioned previously when it comes to communities, it's important not only to make sure that the relationship is reciprocal but also that the other person is actually providing you with the support that you need. Being noticed is great, but it isn't actual support. This might be hard for you to pinpoint right away, especially if you don't tend to need community support from others until something is really wrong. Far be it from me to guess the motivations for people to put themselves in the spotlight of the community by running events or growing a following, but I would be wary about assuming that people are in charge in polyamory communities because they are great partners.

Lack of diverse perspectives

After I stopped going to polyamory community events, I actually ended up meeting more polyamorous people. The biggest difference between the polyamorous people that I met outside and the people that I met inside of 'the community' was a variety of privileges. Most of the people I knew from 'the community' were white and came from middle class backgrounds and/or were middle class themselves. And while there was a decent showing of queer folks, there wasn't a lot of discussion about what queer people experienced.

Eventually I withdrew from my local community. A big reason I stopped wanting to be involved was the lack of diverse perspectives from people both like and different to myself. I witnessed the suggestion that the community wasn't perfect or the idea to focus on something other than polyamory come up countless times, but they would often be pretty brusquely rejected by many people. In some of these situations, there was an attempt at diversifying the perspectives, but usually in a tokenistic way.

Not to mention, when I was trying to compare my life to people in the community, there were things I was facing such as struggles with trying to find work, not having family support, dealing with immigration and coping with my disability that other people just weren't facing. Even something as simple as deciding to stay at someone's house wasn't easy for me because I had medication I needed to take at certain times. I perpetually felt like a wet blanket just because I couldn't do all the other things that people with more access than me could do.

Because I'm white, it's hard for me to address the issue that I noticed in my local community, which was that white people not only dominated most of the community events I attended but also held all the power. I can address it by recognizing and identifying the trend as I saw it, but I can't speak of how difficult it is to not be white and cope with the polyamory community. I noticed that so many people I've met outside of the polyamory community are not white and are also not interested in going to community events, or expressly have noted the struggles they've faced in 'the community' which have not been addressed to enable them to feel safe returning.

Being polyamorous as a commonality, as I've mentioned, is one small thing that binds you together but there are lots of different ways to do polyamory and reasons for being poly-amorous. Being polyamorous itself doesn't represent all your life experiences and all the things that you have to face that will definitely impact your polyamory. I didn't manage to find even white-dominated polyamory perspectives that factored in neurodiversity and mental health issues until almost five or six years after I first discovered polyamory. But it may be that many communities are shifting and things are improving so more of these perspectives are coming out.

So, when you're looking at your local community, ask yourself if people share some of the issues that you're facing in your life and how that impacts your polyamory. While theoretically we should not compare ourselves to others, sometimes that will happen. And when you're reaching out for help and emotional understanding from your community, it might be harder to get that if you're having to explain some basic concepts to the members who might have their own ignorance to work out and can't relate to what you're going through.

If you're not in a polyamory community with at least a few people who reflect your experiences, you may end up feeling like you're the only one struggling, especially if you're coping with mental health issues. If you're more apt to blame yourself, you can mistake what is just other people's inability to understand where you're coming from for the idea that something must be inherently wrong with you.

Identifying abuse

I don't think I've ever really witnessed a community handle accusations of abuse or assault well, so I don't think this is an issue that's solely within polyamory. As I've mentioned, like the BDSM community, a good many people are under the impression or get told that people who behave abusively will be phased out of a community like some sort of weird natural selection. You definitely get told this lie when it comes to the BDSM community – that people who do harm will just be silently excluded and fade into the ether, so there's nothing to worry about.

Unfortunately, this has not been my experience in any community. It's not to say that there aren't some successful efforts to stop people who seem to frequently and carelessly harm others, but there are two main problems with this approach: it relies on the presumption that the person who is abusing others will always be identified clearly and will become unpopular, and it also assumes that shutting abusive people out of the community is the best way to solve the problem every time.

I recommend *Why Does He Do That?* by Lundy Bancroft frequently because a friend encouraged me to read it when I was just starting out in a relationship. Because of my own experience of abuse and my ignorance, I assumed that people who abused others didn't really have control of their faculties and that was a large part of why they abused others. That book helped me understand that, as out of control as people may seem, there is far more to it than that.

Another thing that Bancroft's book highlighted to me was that abusive relationships are rarely all bad and that people who abuse can often be great people when they aren't abusing their partners. It's not as simple as finding a complete monster among angels. People often assume that because polyamory is breaking the tradition that society sets forth with monogamy, it is somehow inherently egalitarian or that they're somehow safe from abuse because everyone who does it is far too enlightened to do that. I see so many things in polyamory communities that reinforce the idea that to be polyamorous, you have to have gone on some type of soul journey or must be an inherently good communicator and none of that is the case. I have argued that polyamory can actually provide a perfect backdrop for abuse and that simply not enough has been written about it for us to identify some of the red flags in polyamory that just might show up differently.

The example I frequently give is that if you are dating someone and all of their other partners claim that they are wonderful and have never hurt them, you're going to doubt yourself even more than you would if you're dating someone and their friends say the person is great. Also, I feel like if you have a partner you see infrequently, then you're less likely to bring up when they are crossing boundaries because you want to take advantage of the time you have together and the time apart may actually help you forget about some of the red flags you've seen.

After I read that book, I started to realize that I didn't have to be grateful for kindness and that it should be a given. I felt more empowered to identify potentially abusive behaviours far earlier than I would have if I hadn't read the book and just assumed there was something wrong with me, especially when I had little experience of polyamory. For the record, I do think that people can have abusive behaviours without being pathologically abusive, especially if they grew up learning abusive behaviours in their background and assuming that is how things are done.

But either way, those behaviours need to be challenged. The assumption that everyone can identify when they are being abused and that they will then be able to identify the person abusing them in order to make effective change isn't really true. Not everyone has the knowledge to realize when this is happening to them. And if someone they're with has a habit of abusing their partners, they are not going to reveal themselves right away. One of the most terrifying stats that I read in the Bancroft book was how frequently men that Lundy Bancroft worked with knowingly didn't begin to get physically abusive with their spouses until they were pregnant.

So, assuming that the community is able to accurately identify people who are either perpetuating abusive behaviours against a partner or are pathologically abusive isn't going to be something that you can rely on. Plus, if you take the previous section on community leaders and popularity into account, you're also going to be coming to grips with what anyone who tries to talk about abuse goes through: the more popular someone is or the more social capital they have, the more likely it is that the people around them will not want to hear anything negative about them. Or, as I say explicitly in one of my articles, if everyone wants to sleep with the person, they're not likely to care what you have to say about them.

Handling abusive behaviour

Again, like with most communities, I haven't seen that the polyamory community knows how to handle abusive behaviours, even when they are identified. I don't think this is because people want to 'hide abusers' or don't care about people who have been abused. I believe that most of us grow up in societies that give us constant messages about what 'justice' is. We're also given many messages about good and evil and usually the punishment for evil is shame, exclusion and humiliation, as we discussed previously regarding making mistakes.

Many of us who grow up either in the slight influence of or directly under the thumb of a fundamentalist belief system that promotes a tortuous afterlife as a punishment for our wrongdoings will be influenced by this as a measure of justice. Even if you grew up in a secular family or society, you might not necessarily see anything wrong with an afterlife of torment – for the right person, at least.

We're not encouraged to have compassion as a part of justice or to see rehabilitation as a viable option. For those of us who have come from abusive backgrounds, being able to have anger at your abuser and actually wish ill upon them are huge steps towards healing. In many cultures, you're encouraged to have something for your abuser that is called compassion and love but is really just silence about your own experiences. Anger is an important step in identifying that something is wrong, but I do think at times we're stuck in anger so much, we feel that anyone who displays abusive behaviour is a monster who is incapable of rehabilitation and can often become a representation of all who have hurt us.

While I don't doubt there are many people out there who are not interested in being rehabilitated, assuming that kicking them out of the community is always the right step creates real problems with power dynamics and exclusion that can actually serve to help rather than hurt abusive people. When we create a system where there are only monsters and heroes, that system can easily be twisted by a person who is abusing someone, especially a person with social power.

If you learn more about abusive pathologies, you start to identify common patterns and one of those is isolating the person they are abusing. Within monogamy, it's in some ways easier to isolate people because you can phase out their friends and family thanks to the cultural assumption that one person should meet all your needs anyway. But within polyamory it's a bit more complicated. I have seen situations where people have been isolated from their communities either because their ex identified them as an 'abuser' online or because people in the community didn't want to associate with an 'abuser' for fear of what it said about them.

There is a lot of discussion online about this phenomenon, especially within left wing or progressive communities, where some call it 'cancel culture'. I personally feel like the phrase 'cancel culture' has adopted a trajectory similar to the phrase 'emotional labour' in that it's been used in so many different ways by so many different people that the who is doing the cancelling to whom changes depending on who is using the word.

Publicized social movements have resulted in more people feeling free to speak about abuse from high-profile people than before, but I'm hesitant to see a for-profit media more willing to cover stories about abuse as progress. I question whether the people with actual large platforms who have been written about have really lost opportunities. And I've also witnessed many people get harassed online for making a mistake that people won't even give them details about and where the only 'accountability' they can take is ceasing to exist.

When we create a system where we chuck people out of a community when they aren't up to snuff, all we do is send that person to another community who may not know about them. I'm not suggesting we adopt a policy where we just allow people to continue to cross boundary after boundary with no confrontation or recognition – but let's be real. That's already the status quo. The only difference is who is forgiven frequently and who is not. We've not even got to a point in most communities where we've established any real agreed upon system of reconciliation, rehabilitation or community healing. It's unsurprising then that people decide to take justice into their own hands.

Most community leaders are not interested in the responsibility of having to decide when to kick someone out or not and will often avoid it. When the choice is only to keep someone or kick them out, then it makes sense that community leaders would be reluctant just to believe anyone who accused anyone, especially if they have a personal experience with the accused. It's hard for me to give an idea of what exactly a restorative and just community would look like because I'm not sure if I should be the one deciding that, but I do know that I don't think that this policy of exclusion is a good way to handle abusive behaviours.

So, when you're going into communities that claim that they have all of this under control, that horrible people are horrible at the core and are promptly shown the door, and everything is safe and perfect, take that with a truckload of salt. There absolutely may be a community out there that has got this all figured out and I've just not come across it. But don't do what I did, which was assume that being in a community that wasn't mainstream was somehow safer. Unfortunately, that's just not the case.

CRABS IN BUCKETS

Being represented within mainstream culture such as films, television or music can sometimes provide you with validation. Within a monogamous-centric society, there is very little in the way of representation of polyamory or non-monogamy in general, and the representation that is available sometimes contributes to the idea that non-monogamy is inherently unstable and a poor choice.

Most people don't necessarily know what 'polyamory' is, but they may be aware of 'open relationships', a relationship status added to Facebook in its early days. No social research has been done to the best of my knowledge, but I don't think it's an unfair assumption that while most people may be aware of open relationships, they think they don't work.

There is a lot to write about visibility and whether or not being accepted into mainstream culture is necessarily a good thing, but suffice to say that the omnipresent idea that open relationships are inherently unstable has a huge impact on a lot of polyamorous people. Some feel like it's more difficult for them to tell family that they are polyamorous than that they are queer.

The result is a mentality that Meg-John Barker points out in their book, *Rewriting the Rules*, which I have also witnessed – the crabs in the bucket. While Meg-John talks about this concept within the context of us being afraid to rewrite our own rules for how relationships go, I think that sometimes when people do venture into polyamory, that same fear of being seen as 'different' and not fitting in added to the fact that polyamory is not mainstream puts people in a position of feeling like they have to prove that open relationships are not inherently unstable, to others and sometimes to themselves.

Power and privilege

I've yet to see any official studies or polls about people's perceptions of 'open relationships' but I wouldn't be surprised if most monogamous people, especially those outside of the queer community, were very adamant that open relationships 'don't work'. People are aware enough of non-monogamy to have a somewhat negative impression of it, but I think the perception of non-monogamous individuals really hinges on other oppressions.

For example, most will judge a woman who has more than one boyfriend very differently than a man who has more than one girlfriend. Many of the examples that people have given me of discrimination against polyamorous people are largely misogynistic discrimination against women. Most of the slurs people have said apply to polyamorous people are misogynistic insults. As more people become culturally aware of polyamory, there may be a shift in that, however I would argue that slurs just aren't about hurt feelings but about social power.

Polyamory and non-monogamy would need to threaten current power dynamics in order to become something that needs to be attacked through a slur. With social marginalization, there is a process by which something is named and identified by the dominant group and stereotyped, dehumanized and ridiculed. There is usually a scapegoating process where this group is blamed for social ills and taught to hate themselves through mainstream culture, which legitimizes physical violence and aggression against them. But within almost every socially marginalized group is a faction of that group that seeks to escape that oppression through assimilation.

In almost every group you will find a person who is dealing with a social marginalization and who feels that most of what they go through is earned due to the ill behaviour of the marginalized. Whether it's victim-blaming women for not behaving in the right way to avoid sexual assault to respectability politics of sagging pants to the hatred of femmes in the gay male community – almost every single group contains those within it who have the desire to assimilate. It's worth noting that we're simplifying social oppressions in this instance and the attribution of intersectionality is incredibly important.

Non-monogamists as a group haven't been studied to the extent that other groups have, so it's hard to pull data about what types of other marginalizations non-monogamous people face that might also mean that non-monogamy only serves to further 'prove' the stereotypes about that individual true. I can say that non-monogamy has been extremely common within the queer community simply because getting married and having kids with a white picket fence was not a realistic goal for many queer people for a very long time.

For many people I've witnessed in the queer community, being non-monogamous is a part of their identity as a queer person. People in the communities I've mentioned that are less likely to be targeted or discriminated against for other reasons (e.g. they are white, middle or upper class, straight, able-bodied, etc.) are more likely to want polyamory to be considered 'normal' and for it not to interrupt any access they may have to other privileges they enjoy.

For those people, proving that non-monogamy 'works' is critical. Showing polyamory as a 'valid' lifestyle is so necessary that it becomes important to emphasize how polyamory is about 'love' and not 'just sleeping around'. It's quite common to run into a lot of attitudes within the polyamory community that reinforce sex negativity, slut-shaming and promote the stigma of sexually transmitted infections, and people wanting to assimilate will be less tolerant of people admitting polyamory is a struggle for them or more willing to declare that people who struggle with polyamory do so because they aren't polyamorous enough.

How many of those people there are in your community who want polyamory to be seen as an 'acceptable' lifestyle with few problems both by outsiders and by themselves will impact how many crabs will be pulling everyone back into the bucket of proving polyamory is 'valid' and thus being less interested in hearing the genuine struggles people have with it.

Doubts and denial

Most polyamory communities online that I've been in are filled with a lot of threads asking for help, which is how I got started giving advice within the community. This isn't all that surprising. The Relationships Reddit channel is not filled with stories of successful monogamous relationships. People are less likely overall to share individual relationship triumphs online with random strangers, especially if they come from cultures that are particularly discouraging of bragging.

We do not judge the success of monogamy by the volume of posts asking for help in the Relationships community on Reddit or in advice columns across the world, but many polyamorous people seem to feel a certain kind of anxiety about the number of posts asking for help or talking about heartbreak in polyamory communities. Almost always I see threads encouraging people to share positive stories, specifically because of the negativity that they witness, whereas very few of those types of posts tend to be found in general relationships communities. No one needs to have it reaffirmed that monogamy can work.

I don't think that everyone who asks to hear positive stories is necessarily concerned with what monogamous people or society at large think, but existing within a culture that doesn't validate your choice of how you want to live your life is going to constantly make you question whether you've made the right choice. Being surrounded by stories of difficulty and heartache, especially those who are giving up polyamory and going back to monogamy, further compounds the issue.

Quite often when you do end up discussing polyamory or non-monogamy with monogamous people, the initial response is how much other people can't do it and questions about jealousy. This means that many polyamorous people don't have a lot of resources or individuals around them to draw from for experiences, reassurance or help, so it's even *more* likely that polyam communities will have a lot of posts asking for help and talking about troubles that people face. The doubt that one 'can do polyamory' accentuates every problem in a way that doesn't occur with monogamy.

All of these combining factors create a perfect storm where a lot of people face a particular pressure to prove outwardly that they can 'do polyamory' or otherwise feel like any problem they may face, especially jealousy, reflects their inability to 'do polyamory'. It's unsurprising that they assume this because a lot of monogamous people think their feelings of jealousy are what's standing between them and trying any form of non-monogamy.

As a result, a lot of people reaching out for help within poly-amory communities might be told outright that they potentially can't 'do polyamory'. Some people may have had partners who pointed out emotions or behaviours as signs that they couldn't 'do polyamory'. Clique-style communities form where people dump on monogamy or create a hierarchical structure where those who can 'do polyamory' are somehow less controlling, more egalitarian, better communicators, healthier and just better people than monogamous people.

People begin to feel vulnerable and anxious about sharing their problems once they are part of a community because they don't want to be seen as a failure at polyamory – or perhaps this is just my experience. At times, some communities seemed divided down the middle: either you have experienced some problems but they are well behind you or something is devastat-ingly wrong. While, again, some communities may be different, I've witnessed this dichotomy in a lot of them. When people talk about the problems they have faced, it's almost always from the perspective of no longer dealing with those problems anymore, of being cured and free from the plague of jealousy through hard work and grit.

Unfortunately, this can become such a pronounced difference that it can seem like jealousy and relationship issues only happen to people who can't 'do polyamory' and that can make people even less likely to reach out for help until it gets dire and repeats this continuous cycle.

Cliques and judgement

One of the things I hate hearing the most when people write into the column is 'monogamy doesn't work'. Whether as a reaction to a monogamous-centric society that's surrounding them, or due to what they read that argues against the conception of monogamy as what's 'natural', or any number of other factors, many communities can devolve into such a crab and bucket mentality and the division can be so entrenched that they can become outright hostile to monogamy.

For many it seems as though the toxic aspects of monogamy are identical to monogamy itself. Particularly when people throw themselves into polyamorous communities and it becomes their primary focus, it can become easier to get wrapped up in a clique bubble. The problem with this, combined with the concept that one can either 'do polyamory' or not, is that it becomes even more difficult to find a place to talk about your problems if the alternative is being part of a community that's seen as inherently harmful and almost less evolved.

While this is another aspect that may vary from community to community, it can be easy to get sucked into the trap of believing that polyamory is the only lifestyle which suits the billions of people on the planet. While I think it's worth exploring the ways we're encouraged to choose monogamy by default and which systems benefit from the specific type of monogamy that society encourages, that doesn't mean monogamy itself is a problem or that polyamory is more natural.

Remember that there is no license (nor do I think there should be) to practise polyamory. Someone being polyamorous doesn't inherently make them any better at communication, handling difficult emotions or holding space for partners who need it, in the same way that a serial monogamist who has dated loads of people isn't necessarily inherently better at any of those things either. Relationships aren't skills themselves and having a lot of them doesn't mean you learned something from each experience.

It can be easy to fall into the trap of assuming that polyamory is 'more difficult' than monogamy. I am not saying that polyamory doesn't come with challenges that are unique and different, but relationships themselves are as varied as the people who are in them. Whether or not something will be challenging for you depends on a lot of factors, some which are out of your control. Polyamory is not a levelled-up version of monogamy and it doesn't require people to be 'better' at relationships to practise – but even I believed that was true at one point.

This is further solidified by some polyamory advice resources, which describe some types of relationships as 'hard level' relationships – such as triads. I have probably also described these types of relationships in that way before, but I am trying to instead describe then as more complex situations. Any relationship can become complex and difficult during certain times, and I think it can be more harmful for others in the long run if we reaffirm the concept that polyamory is 'more difficult' or 'takes more' than monogamy.

One of the biggest results of this is the assumption that can easily form among polyamorous people that nobody in the community is monogamous when it's possible for someone to be monogamous to a polyamorous person. We create communities then where it's more difficult for people to admit when they feel like they're struggling or feel shame if they feel like monogamy is actually what they prefer – which should be just as acceptable as any other choice. Triads also aren't for everyone. That doesn't mean that people who don't want one are too weak to have one.

Coming out of the bucket

One of the best things I've ever read about the phenomenon of how crabs in buckets will pull other crabs back in when they try to get out is this: crabs don't naturally occur in buckets. One of the reasons I like this analogy for many polyamory communities is because, ideally, we would have models or some cultural scripts to follow around us. Whether polyamory is 'accepted' by the 'mainstream' or not, it would be helpful for many if there were some cultural scripts to follow.

Eventually, I do think that things will progress to the point where we will have some cultural scripts for polyamory and then we will exist in an environment that affirms us in similar ways as we're affirmed in monogamy. We won't feel the need to prove ourselves as much and might be much more willing to discuss some of the issues that we're facing on a day-to-day basis without feeling the same amount of shame.

But most of us are unable to immediately change the cultures around us in any large way, so a good way for us to climb out of the bucket is to learn to challenge the way we speak about monogamy as well as be more comfortable with admitting in our communities that we are struggling or that we have problems with 'jealousy' as dreaded as that may seem, and not just when we've 'solved' it or when it's too much to handle. That might be difficult for someone who is new to polyamory or just starting out in the community, but at the very least, keep in mind that others might feel nervous about sharing what they're struggling with.

If you have the privilege of being able to take an active role in the community nearer to you, make sure it's a place where people can feel welcome regardless of whether they lean towards monogamy or polyamory, challenge attitudes that suggest that polyamorous people are more evolved, acknowledge the privileges that people in your group have and seek to find ways that people can get involved in the decision-making process of the groups regardless of what types of commitments they have in their life.

Take conflict management courses or learn about nervous system regulation. It would be ideal if the people who lead communities know how to mediate situations to bring about compromise. Read about transformative and restorative justice and how to challenge your own assumptions about what justice means. Even if you aren't or can't be a community leader, sometimes having just one person to encourage someone not to assume that they're somehow 'bad at polyamory' because they have feelings is beneficial and helpful overall.

POWER IMBALANCES

All relationships contain some power imbalances. This can be caused by wider systems that surround us and also by our personal individual experiences. Imbalances can be the result of situations, such as if you have a partner who lives with another partner and doesn't live with you. It's important to have real conversations in relationships about the power dynamics that might affect the relationship and try to avoid getting defensive. It's also important to realize that while one might *feel* helpless, there is a lot we can do to address our feelings and mindset to escape that feeling of helplessness.

This may be a difficult discussion to have with a partner who doesn't acknowledge or recognize social systems that affect marginalized identities, but it's still worth having. One might say that if a person isn't really willing to recognize how affected you can be by these systems, they may not make for the best partner. They should be at least willing to see how you individually are impacted, even if they're not able to address wider systemic issues.

In the space below, write out the main ways you feel disempowered:

. . . .

. . . .

. . . .

What steps, if any, can your partners take to address this?

. . . .

. . . .

. . . .

What steps, if any, can you take to address this disempowerment?

. . . .

. . . .

. . . .

How do you see these imbalances affecting your relationships?

. . . .

. . . .

. . . .

How might these power imbalances change over time?

. . . .

. . . .

. . . .

COMMUNITY SUPPORT
AND PRIVACY

It's important to recognize that we may reach out to our communities for help if we need it, but we must make sure that we respect the privacy of the people involved in our relationships. Sometimes, people don't really think about the privacy of the people involved until some type of boundary has been crossed. You should always be able to talk to someone about your relationship and if you have a partner who never wants you to seek out any help with your relationship, this isn't a good sign.

However, it's good to discuss and think about whom you would talk to about your problems and what issues may arise from that. Complete the following questions here or in a journal prompt and, if it's helpful, share them with partners.

Who do I have to rely on in and outside of my community?

. . . .

. . . .

. . . .

Who do I expect my partner(s) may rely on for help in or outside of their community?

. . . .

. . . .

. . . .

Are there specific details I would not like shared with others?

. . . .

. . . .

. . . .

What are my main concerns with relying on members of my community?

. . . .

. . . .

. . . .

What Will You Do?

∞

After you start getting involved in communities or doing more reading, you may begin to have some of your first non-monogamous relationships. You've already considered your ideals and your worst fears, whom you might rely on, and what power imbalances may be in play when you set out. Some of these are subject to change and it's always worth reviewing them further down the line.

This chapter will focus on some of the more tangible, planning aspects of non-monogamy.

SCHEDULING AND TIME

If you've already considered your ideal setup, then you are one step ahead of where a lot of people can find themselves when starting off in polyamory or non-monogamy. Especially if you're already dating someone monogamously and you plan on 'opening up', one of the biggest things that I think people fail to do, which creates more difficulty in accepting the shift in lifestyles, is immediately consider ways to rearrange their time and schedules.

Spent time is not dedicated time

In some instances, when two people 'open up' they won't act very differently to how they did monogamously, which is why I think so many people think they can agree to non-monogamy without fundamentally changing how their relationship is set up – because for many, if their partner spends the same amount of time around them and with them, not much has actually changed for them right away. I think it can also make it much harder when those first nights without your partner happen, because you're not only having something new happen, which is your partner being away from you, but you're also having to deal with a new aspect of them being away.

If you're living together, you can also quite easily assume that time spent *around* one another is time spent *with* one another and therefore it can be easier to feel like your partner is going out of their way to spend time with others rather than with you. It's important to consider not just time spent away but also intentional time spent with partners that you live with.

It's also worth thinking about how you want to spend time dedicated to each other and whether it is spent on a mutually enjoyable activity – or whether or not there is enough compromise within the relationship to figure out whether one person is giving too much to the other. Actively thinking about the time you spend together can also help work through some of the issues, if there are any, in current relationships and identify where there might be imbalances that are building resentment that need to be addressed before they get larger and become a real issue.

This is also a good opportunity to consider what represents time dedicated for you. Some people may feel like they don't need their partner's full attention and others may enjoy more alone time. Dedicated time may be when you decide to put all distractions aside to focus on the task at hand or one another. Setting some ground rules for, barring emergencies, how we operate during dedicated time before it becomes an unmet need can address issues before they become bigger problems.

Changing plans

Another aspect that might be equally challenging is deciding when is 'too soon' to change plans or shift schedules. If you're on the autistic spectrum like me or struggle with abandonment fears, sudden schedule changes could create a lot more anxiety, which can be easy to mistake for jealousy. Even if the schedule change is understandable, it can still create worries that need to be addressed.

Some partners may be able to cope with sudden schedule changes better than others, so it's always worth factoring that in when you're talking about scheduling. Without understanding that this could be an issue, not factoring it in could mean trying to figure out if you're upset because plans changed or because you're assigning more meaning to the schedule change than there is.

To figure out if a scheduling issue is due to feeling negative or unhappy with a metamour, jealousy or just an issue with the scheduling itself, I always ask myself whether I would be upset if two friends did the same.

So, for example, I found myself snapping at my partner and metamour when they had some alone time after I had been waiting outside in the cold and was in pain all day. There was a miscommunication and I had been waiting for an hour already for them because I was confused about when they were leaving, so I was already frustrated. I would have probably been just as snappy with two friends who had done the same. It wasn't at all about the partner involved, just about me being cold and grumpy, but handling the situation the way I did made my metamour feel like they had done something wrong.

Miscommunications and misunderstandings will happen. Plans might shift and change. Sometimes dates may go really well and you may not want them to end. Work and other obligations pop up. It's important to give people space to be frustrated with that but also know when the right time is to express those frustrations and own up to how you do express them. Identify which plans are flexible and which plans can be changed only in an emergency.

Also think about how and when to address situations as they arise. If you know that you experience some anxiety when plans suddenly change, having other people to rely on and talk to whenever you're going through some of these emotions is important. Give yourself the space to just feel and have a place to express that feeling without picking it apart immediately.

Having read the previous chapters on jealousy or insecurity, you might be able to pinpoint what the underlying issue is and how best to address it and whether or not it makes sense to address it right when the plans change or later on when the dust settles.

Flexibility shifts

Your flexibility when it comes to meet ups might also change as your trust builds. When you're just opening up or you're starting a new relationship, you're building trust and part of that is honouring your word with someone. When you cancel or change things last minute during that trust-building stage, it can be a bit harder for the other person to weather it.

Especially if they face mental health struggles, it can be difficult for people to sit through these changes without allowing self-doubt to creep in or wondering if this is like another situation they may have experienced where someone lost interest but didn't want to be honest. But as you start to build trust (whether it's a new relationship or changing a current one), you'll feel a little less anxious when things change. And if you're just starting out in non-monogamy, having a partner cancel something with you to spend time with a new partner can be difficult to experience without assigning extra meaning to it.

This actually is fairly true for monogamy as well – people get anxious when dates cancel on them. We just have a cultural script to reassure us when things like this happen. There is a certain amount of sitting in discomfort when plans have to be shifted or changed, but you can also solve this by scheduling time not just away from a partner but also *with* them. Ensuring that there is adequate time scheduled with all partners is important.

This is another situation where recognizing what you can or can't control can help adapt to some of the anxiety around changing plans and being flexible. If you have a partner who is not going to prioritize you in terms of their time, who won't spend dedicated time with you and who continues to show you through cancelling dates that they don't care about you, there is little you can do to change that from a scheduling standpoint. If you have a better idea of expectations and your needs, it can keep you from spiralling into anxiety when things like plan changes happen and can also encourage you to state your needs and find out earlier if you have a partner who is not meeting them.

Taking responsibility for time

Equally, it's also important to take responsibility for the decisions you make about your time once you have multiple schedules to balance. Too many times I see people either trying to please everyone to the point where they overschedule, or they get so caught up in new relationship energy, they don't seem to pay as much attention to their decisions as they normally would.

Whether you believe in practising non-hierarchical forms of non-monogamy or not, your scheduling and timing can speak louder than your principles. And you can easily *believe* you have a non-hierarchical approach but then schedule your time in very hierarchical ways. And absolving yourself of responsibility for your own schedule by giving it to another partner to handle isn't taking responsibility for your time and isn't fair to any of your partners.

This is where things can get difficult for people who have had problems with setting their own boundaries or who really struggle with the concept of disappointing or letting down partners. Making decisions about how you choose to spend your time may come with some disappointments in the same way navigating any busy schedule might. It's one of the main aspects of managing your relationships and sometimes it might involve being really honest with yourself about your capacity and time and also learning that your partners may be disappointed but that doesn't mean they dislike you.

Within the polyamory community, people frequently say 'love is infinite' but I constantly remind people in the column and podcast that time is not infinite. We only have 24 hours in a day and so much energy to spend in those hours. The amount of privilege we have can also dictate how we're best able to use that time. In addition to romantic relationships, we also have friendships, family, work, hobbies and everything else to manage within that time period.

Originally, I struggled with the concept of not having a hierarchy because of my disability. There have been times when adjusting to medication where I have barely had the energy to work and shop for food, where I'd not be able to date because I'd need to collapse as soon as I got home to take a nap in order to have the energy to make dinner. And before that, I had been living with my parents, unable to drive and working three jobs. In both of those situations it felt impossible to sustain even a single romantic relationship, let alone multiple ones.

As things have changed in my life, I've realized I have more capacity than I assumed I had, but I'm also better able to understand what kinds of relationships I've got capacity for. I've been able to help friends and devote time to them when I've needed to, even while dealing with difficult personal things on my own. Our capacity doesn't always remain the same as our lives change.

It's okay to misunderstand your own capacity and to want to have more romantic relationships than you can realistically manage. Sometimes the needs that other people have within relationships can shift in the same way that they do outside of romantic relationships and what was once something you could manage changes into something you can't. Being responsible for your time doesn't mean that you necessarily always know when something becomes 'too much', but that you communicate it as early as possible instead of waiting until it becomes intolerable for the other people.

Scheduling separate time

When you're first starting out, especially if you're living with a partner, it might aid the transition to schedule time apart and time together even if it feels ridiculous or unnecessary. You don't necessarily have to spend time dating or trying to find a partner in your scheduled time apart – even having separate hobbies you can pursue on your own time can work.

Equally, scheduling time together is also important whether it's a date night once a week or planned meals together. Intentional time apart and intentional time together will help it become a little bit easier when there are other people in the mix because it will allow trust to build in scheduling and, especially if you live together, honouring agreements with one another. It will feel less jarring overall when someone is spending time with someone else if you already have experience of them doing more things on their own and it will make it easier to cope with.

This is actually something I would also advise monogamous people who live together to do. Again, just because you spend time *around* one another doesn't mean you're spending time *with* one another and one of the unfortunate side effects of following the relationship escalator is that intentional time often gets lost in the mix, hobbies and other relationships get dulled down, and often things become monotonous. It also might explain why so many struggle when their partners die. Keeping some independence even within monogamy could be beneficial for keeping monogamous relationships alive as well.

EMERGENCIES

When an emergency involves a life-or-death situation, it feels a lot easier for us to prioritize. But non-life-or-death situations can still be emergencies. The more people involved in your dynamic, the more complicated protocol for emergencies can become. Thinking about some of these incidents before they happen can make your decision process a little bit simpler and clearer.

Priorities and choices

In a lot of my earlier polyamory writings, I was pretty negative towards the concept of relationship anarchy, because the people I'd met and examples I'd been shown who were supposedly practising relationship anarchy were really just using it as a way to avoid responsibility for decisions about how they spent their time and the impact it had on partners. It felt like 'relationship anarchy' was a shorthand to get out of any emotional responsibility in any relationship. But I was wrong. I consistently also misunderstood the concept of non-hierarchical relationship approaches.

For me, it didn't make sense that I would consider someone I just met as important as someone I'd known for ten years and I think that was an extreme example. When I lost some of the important friendships in my life, I finally realized just how much friendships meant to me and that I didn't necessarily see romantic relationships as inherently more important than close friendships, just different. I also had to accept the realization that just because someone has been in my life for a long time doesn't mean they necessarily care more about me or are more trustworthy than someone who just became my friend.

We're not often forced to think about the priorities we'd make until the absolute worst happens and then it seems more obvious, but within polyamory and especially if you want to practise a more anti-hierarchical style where you consider all of your relationships as equally important, handling emergencies becomes slightly more complex.

How to define an 'emergency'

It's worth thinking about what kinds of emergencies might come up with all the types of relationships you have in your life and how you might respond to them. This plays partially into the concept of your ideal polyamory setup. Having an ideal where you have ten partners may sound great at first, but what sort of emotional responsibility do you have towards all ten of those people, as well as the rest of the people in your life? What type of relationships do you want with your metamours and how involved will you be?

Once you begin to see your ideal polyamory set up through the lens of also providing support to the individuals involved, it may shift what you consider an 'ideal' and it might be worth revisiting and revising your 'ideal'. This isn't to say you're going to be able to prepare yourself for every potential issue or problem – far from it. But having a good understanding of what kind of response you might make in emergencies might help you have a good understanding of the support network you have, what your responsibilities are and what expectations you have.

Emergencies that aren't immediately obvious (e.g. someone in a hospital) might include: having a non-life-threatening mental health crisis, a death in the family, breaking up with another partner, dropping out of school, losing a job, failing a test, moving to a new town, etc. Any major life event that might shake up someone's established sense of security can be something that partners can help emotionally with. These are also things that friends can respond to. We might cancel a date we have with our partner if our best friend's father passed away suddenly, for example.

Not all these situations would be classed as a direct 'emergency', but they are still sudden events that may require support from people's immediate circle. People can have all different types of partnerships and being a partner to someone doesn't necessarily mean you're part of the immediate circle they rely on, but it's better that you both know that instead of them expecting your support during a hard time and not being able to get it.

Expectations and responsibility

We often don't think about our plans for these types of situations because the cultural script of monogamy gives a basic type of hierarchy that tends to work – although I would note that many relationship advice columns are filled with questions about whether or not someone is too close to a friend or whether or not someone should have to be around an abusive in-law. Even those scripts that are given don't work for every monogamous life – so why would they work in a life where there are even more people to manage?

Having a bit of an idea of what you might do in the case of different emergencies and having a discussion on what to expect in each case, what you're responsible for and what your partners' expectations are can be incredibly helpful for thinking through things in the future. Some partners may need more emotional support than others. Some may need emotional support right away or much later.

Once you have something more established together, expectations of support may change. It might be worth going through with partners what types of emergency situations they have been through before and what support they have needed in the past. It also might be worth revisiting these every once in a while to make sure you're able to see how things have changed and shifted throughout time.

CHECK-INS AND CHECK-UPS

Too often people make the mistake of only checking in on partners when they think something may be wrong, when they have something to disclose, or they make rules like 'you have to tell me when you have feelings for people'. There's an ongoing joke about how polyamorous people over-communicate and I think that can be true to a certain extent, but when you're starting out in opening a relationship or going out on dates with new partners, sometimes more communication can be helpful to establish trust.

Because it's not such a common practice within monogamy, it isn't something that comes naturally to most people. Relationship discussions are usually done within monogamy when something serious and negative happens, or when there is a massive change. Learning to practise discussion regularly can help individuals involved learn to address issues without being immediately set on high alert just because a discussion is taking place.

When you have feelings

One of the most common mistakes people make when they open their relationship is making a rule that their partner will let them know when they 'start to have feelings for someone else'. There are two main problems with this: it assumes that everyone has enough awareness to realize when their feelings are at a certain level or that everyone has the same definition of what makes a feeling worth noting, and it also assumes that something can be prevented by letting your partner know when you begin to have feelings about someone.

This rule is designed to encourage regular communication about when there might be changes to the way the relationship is currently progressing, but in reality you don't need to create a rule like that in order to communicate consistently. We must also remember that, as silly as this may sound, growing up in a monogamous-centric society encourages us to be emotionally hardwired to believe that having feelings for someone else is an inherent threat to our relationship, even if we technically have permission to do so.

Though it seems confusing and counterintuitive, many people find it easier to cheat than to be honest with their partner and end up accidentally cheating just because they don't know when to disclose a feeling or a relationship building. Or, even if they haven't felt like they've cheated, because their partner is more aware of their behaviours than they are, their partner can feel cheated on and gaslit because they *see* their partner behaving as if they are dating someone else, but they haven't been told officially that 'the Feelings' have arrived.

We all have our own subjective emotional experience and, as much as part of our society encourages us to believe it's possible for a human being to be completely objective or to apply criteria objectively, I find it more useful to remember this quote from Edward Said in *Orientalism*:

> No one has ever devised a method for detaching the scholar from the circumstances of life, from the fact of [their] involvement (conscious or unconscious) with a class, a set of beliefs, a social position, or from the mere activity of being a member of a society.

From the outset, we're encouraged to see romantic relationships as 'more than friends' without us really knowing what it means exactly when you 'have feelings' for someone or that this experience is necessarily shared by everyone. The biggest reason why there is a cultural script in monogamy is to define different stages of a relationship's 'progression' into what is supposed to be something more 'stable' and 'committed'.

When we abandon those scripts, it becomes less clear what it means to 'have feelings' for someone or how to define a relationship's 'progression' (or if it needs to 'progress'). For many people, 'having feelings' means increasing your expectations of the relationship and someone else's emotional commitment to you, which is often expressed by a desire for exclusivity. If you don't have a desire for exclusivity, then where does that leave you? If 'having feelings' refers to a sexual and romantic attraction, but people can have sexual and romantic attractions to friends without the expectation of any kind of 'commitment', where does that leave you?

These are things people often don't consider before making this rule and then, when they find themselves in the middle of something, end up confused as to what and when they're meant to tell their partner. Especially when this rule is coupled with promises like, 'I'll never love anyone as much as you' or 'No one will ever replace you', it becomes even more confusing because there is now a baseline of feeling that you are promising that you can't even control.

And then, if you make a mistake and don't communicate at the precise time you're meant to, you can end up accidentally breaking this rule and the consequences of 'cheating' are then also defined by our experience of cheating in monogamy, which is usually characterized as a deliberate action. At times, the definition of an action as 'cheating' when it doesn't have to be defined that way causes more harm because of the emotional weight that 'cheating' carries with it rather than just the emotional weight of the action itself.

Rather than making this rule, communicating regularly about how you're feeling about the relationship and your other relationships makes for a better goal, especially towards the beginning of the relationship or when opening the relationship and building trust with each other. Instead of trying to predict or prevent change, expect that change will happen and focus on how you will work together to regularly address it.

Connection not prevention

Initially discussions can help you build a good connection with your partner and provide a good space to air concerns and worries, but it's important to remember that not everything can be solved or prevented by conversation. If you have a fundamental incompatibility, there's only so much that you can do to solve it through a discussion.

Discussion also can only do so much to prevent future problems from happening. All relationships throughout time have some form of conflict and it's important that, rather than avoiding all conflict, you know what happens when you have a disagreement and come to a resolution together. I made the mistake earlier in my relationships of assuming that having no conflict at all meant the relationship was going well and, while some relationships may have less conflict than others, if you end up avoiding all conflict, it causes problems that will come out eventually and often more intensely.

The point of regular discussions should be connecting and providing a space for you to talk about the relationship, the positives as well as the negatives. This doesn't necessarily have to be formalized or happen at specified times. You could do this with a professional or do it on your own. If you have a triad or quad dynamic, this might be extremely helpful in making sure that you're addressing the relationship dynamic that exists between everyone present rather than only as sets of individuals.

Making regular time for a discussion about ongoing issues or feelings can help build trust and provide an easy space for reassurance. It can also increase your tolerance for discussing more serious things if you discuss things that make you happy as well as things you want to work on. It's definitely going to be odd at first because, as aforementioned, this isn't something that's typically done in monogamy until there are very serious problems. The first few meetings are likely to be nerve-wracking or weird, but it's worth getting used to regularly talking instead of expecting a rule to do that for you.

When it comes to your personal dynamic, work out what works for you and each partner. One approach won't necessarily work for every single person or relationship dynamic. Definitely consider regular relationship discussions as an option because it's not something many people assume can be done when they are raised within a monogamous-centric culture. Using rules to indirectly create security sometimes creates more problems than it solves.

Disclosure and awkwardness

There's no way around this and I've not felt any different about it in the near decade that I've been officially polyamorous – disclosure is very awkward and feels a bit strange. Even if you don't have a rule where a partner has to tell you when they have feelings for someone else, you may have a rule about being notified about any change in STI risk status. Even if disclosure is a little bit more straightforward and not as nerve-wracking, it's still sometimes awkward.

As I've mentioned before, disclosing to your partner that you are interested in or have already had sex with someone else is essentially where the rubber meets the road. While regular discussion practices might make you feel a little less nervous overall about discussing things, it's very understandable to have a good amount of anxiety the first time you feel like there's something you want to disclose.

It's worth thinking about and discussing with your partners when it might be ideal to disclose STI risk in particular. One of the examples I've always given to people when they have the rule that their partners *must* tell them *before* having any sexual contact with anyone else is a partner out at a party deciding that they want to sleep with someone and trying to get you on the phone or a messaging service in the middle of a night when you've had insomnia and a lot of stress from work. While that rule sounded excellent when you were discussing it, the actual practice of it might end up creating more problems.

There is a difference in my relationships between someone hiding something from me and someone deciding to choose to disclose something to me when they know I am in a better state to receive it. The shooting that happened in the club in Orlando had a huge impact on LGBTQ communities both in the US and abroad and, when it happened, my mental health on the day and days after wasn't great. My partner at the time chose to wait to disclose a change in STI risk (which they knew based on our rules wasn't going to change the protection we used with each other) until I had mentally recovered from dealing with the tragedy.

There may be times in your life, especially if you struggle with mental health ups and downs, where, while disclosure may be important, in the moment it may end up being more harmful than good. Deciding when to hold disclosure during an emergency or tragedy can be tricky. Sometimes it can seem more like a partner is avoiding disclosure if they have done something that they know may trigger a mental health dip because they don't want to have to bear the emotional responsibility of their actions – and I have certainly seen examples of people who have done so. But at the same time, your partner may also not always have the mental health resources themselves to support you through what their disclosure might bring up at the moment and may want to wait until they do.

Sometimes there aren't easy answers in more complicated situations. While what my partner did during the aftermath of the Orlando shooting made sense to me individually, it may have not worked well for someone else or it may not work well for me in other situations. Different situations might call for different disclosure practices and one size may not fit all situations. It's important to recognize though that, unless there is a general overall pattern of avoiding your emotional needs, a partner who avoids an immediate disclosure isn't necessarily 'cheating' or hiding anything – they just may be trying to balance your needs with their own.

Talking with each other about what to disclose, how to disclose it and what to do in situations of mental or physical health challenges is worth thinking about before they arise and make things difficult. Some people may find it easier to cope with the awkwardness of disclosure by texting about it, rather than talking. It may be that the process of disclosing is what leads someone to recognize that polyamory is not for them. In the first couple of experiences of disclosure, especially if you grew up in a monogamous-centric culture, you may find your feelings going from grounded to chaos to grounded again.

You're never going to be able to prepare for every single emotional eventuality, but it's worth considering times when you have received bad news (and also good news) in your life and how you have coped with that in the past. Sometimes you may not know you have a boundary or a preference until it's been crossed or not followed – and that doesn't necessarily have to mean any malicious intent on the part of the partner who crossed it. Trying to work through some of these difficulties may only truly happen when you're face to face with them.

Reassurance and asking for help

One of the key issues that a lot of people find when they are starting out and going on dates with new people is concern about how to reassure their partner when they are out or, in the opposite position, how and when to ask for reassurance when a partner is with someone else. Opening your relationship or trying a new relationship style comes with a certain level of anxiety, but it can absolutely be difficult to tell if this anxiety is 'bad enough' to warrant reaching out, especially if the anxiety you already have leaves you feeling frustrated with yourself and exasperated. And what makes it even worse is what counts as 'bad enough' isn't really knowable by anybody but the individual experiencing the anxiety and it's not always easy to tell.

Some people decide to make rules around how frequently their partners must contact them during dates or try to establish a level of constant contact with their partner. While often rules like this get interpreted as controlling (and certainly partners can make controlling rules that look exactly like this), sometimes they are just an effort to have a guaranteed method of reassurance because they find it difficult to tolerate the uncertainty while their partner is away. During the earlier stages of my partnership, I've asked, but not demanded, that if my partner has time while they are staying overnight somewhere, I would love to have a goodnight call. As my partner spent more time away and our trust with each other grew, I have felt like I needed this less and less.

However, it's not realistic and not really even fair for your partner to take out time from focusing on another partner to focus on you – even if you're struggling to cope on your own. That may come off as harsh, especially when you're finding it particularly distressing that your partner is away or if you have to be the one to establish that communication boundary. When I'm wondering how to judge an issue and work with my thought process – not to find who is at fault, but to figure out whether my response to a certain situation is coming from a place of my fear of being replaced – I will often think about how I would feel if my partner were visiting a family member or, if they had a child, spending time with their child.

Would I expect someone who was spending time with their child to text me multiple times throughout their day as a rule? Would I make that rule if they were spending time with their family instead of going on a date? Or with a group of friends? This is where someone who has a desire to control their partner would expect constant access to them, regardless of whom they are with. You might say that you wouldn't have as much anxiety if your partner were just visiting a friend. And that may be true.

The key difference between visiting a family member and going on a date is the fear of change and losing your partner – and that's where reassurance from your partner actually *isn't* going to work in the long term.

Reassurance is an important part of any relationship and even people who would claim to be incredibly mentally healthy may go through bouts of difficulty and need reassurance from partners, friends and loved ones. As aforementioned in the section on independence, we're not individual islands and we function well when we have others around us who can help bring us back to a stasis and help support us. This is one of the reasons why people behaving abusively seek to isolate their victims. However, like anything else, there can become a point, not necessarily where we are relying on reassurance too much, but where we're expecting reassurance to solve something it can't.

Those who have struggled with poor mental health or have a history of abuse may struggle with the idea that their needs are not reasonable or even worth asking for. Before I learned how to state my needs, I would often, instead of directly asking, try to manipulate situations so that I got what I needed without *having to ask directly.* I distinctly remember a time when I needed my partner's company because I was dealing with mourning, but they were heading to a party. I kept offering to cook for them or watch their favourite shows to entice them over, but they wanted to go to the party. I was too afraid to ask directly and I found myself starting to get upset. My partner, in their wisdom, instead of reacting to me getting upset defensively, simply asked me if I needed them. When I said that I did, they skipped the party and came to see me.

Learning how to be okay with asking for help was not easy for me. Admitting that I needed something from someone else has historically not been a good idea for me, so I learned that it was better just not to be that vulnerable. And while that may have served me well at some points in my life, within partnerships it meant that I wouldn't ask for what I needed and when I caught myself feeling vulnerable and sad, I would get angry in response as a defence mechanism.

Growing up my only options were not to need anything or to demand it angrily so as to prevent myself being mocked, so that was my go-to as an adult in relationships. If I had not had the partner I had, who didn't take my upset personally and was willing to work with me when they recognized I was hurt and scared, I likely would have continued this pattern for much longer. And this is one of the best examples I have of when partnerships can have a healing effect and help you do more work than you can necessarily do on your own.

Negotiating reassurance

The benefit of me not wanting to ask for help, however, was that I usually would try to find other solutions for resolving my anxiety when my partner was away so I didn't have to rely on reassurance. While it wasn't necessarily healthy to feel like I couldn't ask for reassurance, the result was that I turned inward and began trying to question the assumptions I made behind my fear. If we are afraid of losing our partners and afraid we are inherently not good enough for anybody, no amount of reassurance from any partner will fix that. Reassurance can be a temporary relief in times when we doubt ourselves, but a partner cannot be a stand-in for your own self-esteem.

I tell people trying polyamory for the first time to expect anxiety, because trying something new will cause anxiety. So many people respond to this with a large amount of reassurance, sometimes with forms of reassurance that just aren't helpful or actually hurt more, instead of focusing on the actual problem, which is the fear and discomfort and learning to sit with it. Many people rely on the short-term boost of reassurance that may eventually become unsustainable. Typically, unhelpful reassurance, as I've mentioned before, looks like 'I love you more than I love anyone else' or even things like, 'Other people mean nothing to me compared to you', which just reaffirms that there is one winner's seat that someone can occupy in your partner's life and you may be in it now, but you could be replaced.

The first step when either asking for reassurance during a time when your partner is with others, or creating boundaries around giving reassurance, is to think about the situation in comparison to other relationships. If there were an emergency like a death in the family or something else where you needed to interrupt your partner, it wouldn't matter who they were with and the situation would have gone beyond just fearing the loss of your partner. If, however, your feelings are stemming from your partner being on a date and fearing the loss or change, it would then be helpful to try and challenge your own fears, as we've discussed previously.

At times, I've found it helpful to do some self-reassurance by, instead of obsessing about how I can compare to the other person, focusing on the positives and benefits that my relationship with my partner brings to my life. I do this by writing letters to my partner about what I'm grateful for in our relationship and about our positive memories. While the common advice is to have a date of your own or a friend over when your partner is out with someone else, when both of these options haven't been possible for me, writing letters has been incredibly useful. Equally, relying on other relationships like friendships to give you reassurance is another way to cope with some of the initial discomfort. Review the primary chapters on finding your 'anchor' as this should also be a way of self-soothing during difficult times.

However, there still may be times when you feel like you need a little extra help with reassurance, especially starting out. Working together to form a compromise – with an exception that this might not happen if the person who is out is very busy – might be something that can help temporarily. The partner who is looking for a balance between respecting the individual they are on a date with and the partner at home may also benefit from comparing the situation to another type of relationship.

If you were on a date and a friend texted you, depending on the type of date, you may shoot a text back, but you may not stop the date to step away and give them a call, unless there was a serious situation they needed your help with.

When forming a compromise on either side, it's important to consider the feelings of the individual on the date with your partner and to respect the time they have with your partner (especially if your partner lives with you). Imagine yourself in that position and consider what you would want from your partner if you were out on a date. This can be very individual. I have friendships where we can be out eating together and both on our phones while casually chatting. Whereas some people make a rule when out for dinner with friends that the first person who looks at their phone pays for the whole tab. Discuss with *all* parties what their preferences are for contact while on dates and remain flexible. Emergencies happen, both physical and mental, and even if you were monogamous you may interrupt a date with your partner to call a friend who was having a crisis or send a text to let them know you'll be there for them later on. There isn't one right way to make an agreement on reassurance, but ensuring that everyone can compromise on something that works for them and that you remain able to soothe yourself in difficult moments are equally important aspects that go into making a compromise work.

If you do not want your partner to spend a lot of time without you, the distress you feel while a partner is gone may only continue to grow despite reassurance given or self-soothing techniques. If you're starting out and worried that you're not 'really polyamorous' because you feel distress, it might help you to recognize that there are things you can do to address that distress and, if polyamory isn't something that works for you, there isn't going to be a secret to addressing that distress that is magically going to change that. So, I would try as many of these techniques as possible over time and see if that helps. If it doesn't, it's possible that polyamory just isn't for you – and that's okay!

SEXUAL HEALTH CHECKLIST

The push to encourage people to use condoms to prevent both pregnancy and the spread of STIs was once called 'safe sex'. STIs were once called STDs. We now say STIs and 'safer sex' for a lot of different reasons, but what I think this illustrates is that there isn't necessarily an agreed definition of what makes something 'safe'. In fact, in many countries, there's been a lot of specific misinformation about particular STIs, such as the herpes simplex virus (HSV).

Many of us have not grown up experiencing age-appropriate sexual health education and so many people do not have a good understanding of STI risk and what to do to protect against it, but shame around the discussion of STIs and catching an STI definitely is more common. I would encourage everyone to have a better understanding of sexual health, but one of the most important discussions to have when you're changing your risk of exposure to an STI is to have a good understanding of what you consider risky.

As an immunocompromised person with a disability that requires constant, exhausting admin, I'm not that keen to add to my current medical diagnosis and complications. This means that I may not be willing to take the same risks my partners may want to. Also, being on the asexual spectrum and just not enjoying the company of most human beings, I just plain don't have much interest in casual sex or sex with people I don't know very well, but I have had partners who do have interest in that. Neither approach is more right nor moral than the other.

In the past, I have been guilty of assuming my comfort level and precautions were a more responsible way of behaving and that partners I had who did not adopt these same precautions or feel the way I did about risk were being foolish or ignorant. It can be easy, especially if you can't personally empathize with what drives people to have an interest in casual sex, to pass judgement on people who engage in behaviours that would feel too risky for you personally. When you negotiate your sexual health risk with others, it's important to remember that there is no one right or superior level of comfort with risk.

It's important to investigate your own assumptions about STIs that have been stigmatized, such as HIV and HSV. While it's understandable if you're in a position like mine not to want another health condition to manage, there are lots of different ways to be sexually intimate with people even if you're a person with a compromised immune system. I have experience working in two ways: with a fluid bonded partner where we had shared rules about the level of risk we would take with new partners and with a partner where we practised as much risk prevention as possible together so that my partner could negotiate their own risk level outside of our relationship as individual scenarios arose. I've found the latter the easiest in terms of managing my anxiety.

No sex is completely risk free and even if you never had sex with another human being, there could always be a risk of contracting STIs from medical equipment that has not been sanitized properly or exposure to someone else's bodily fluids through trauma or attack. We understand when we drive or get into a car that there is a risk of a car crash, but we consider the benefits of transportation to be worth it. Just as we question the assumptions of what we can control when we have fears about our relationships, equally we should question what we assume we can control when we have fears about our STI exposure.

I remember clearly once trying to get my partner to accept a shared rule that they would only have sex with someone they had known for a few months and them outright challenging me that STI risk does not change based upon how well you know someone nor does an STI behave differently based on the attitude of different people. Consider what assumptions you might be making about STI safety that might be less embedded in the science of the risk and more embedded in the sexual shame that many cultures encourage people to have for having an STI.

You may have great local sexual health information on your government website or local charities. If you're not sure where to look, I have recommended the Scarleteen website for a long time. Even if it's specifically for American teenagers, it still might be helpful for you as an adult because the emphasis is on educating people at a variety of reading levels in a direct and relatable way.

These questions have been arranged to help you come up with your comfort level in terms of risk. I would encourage you to fill this out, set some time aside to learn about STIs and then answer the questions again. You could answer these questions now and then come back later in six months and answer them again. See how your comfort levels change, even if the actual STIs themselves have not. While STIs do have mutations, generally speaking, how they spread and your general risk based on activity does not change.

How often do you get tested for STIs and why?

. . . .
. . . .
. . . .

When you get tested for STIs, which ones do you get tested for and why?

. . . .
. . . .
. . . .

Did you know that getting 'tested for STIs' doesn't mean getting tested for all STIs in some clinics?

. . . .
. . . .
. . . .

What precautions do you take with your current partners and why?

....
....
....

What do you find yourself most afraid of contracting (including pregnancy) and why?

....
....
....

How would you/have you disclosed an STI to a previous partner and/
or a new partner and why?

....
....
....

How do you/would you, if you had an STI, prevent a new or current
partner from contracting it and why?

....
....
....

What sexual activities do you consider the most risky and why?

....
....
....

How have your safer sex practices changed throughout time and why?

. . . .

. . . .

. . . .

If someone disclosed to you that they had an STI, what would you do and why?

. . . .

. . . .

. . . .

Are there any barriers that you feel prevent you from accessing sexual healthcare?

. . . .

. . . .

. . . .

What messages, if any, did you get about STIs growing up and what opportunities have you been given to learn more or unlearn this information?

. . . .

. . . .

. . . .

If working through these answers with a partner, it might be useful to write down some points or complete answers on your own and then reconvene together and talk through each of the points. Once you have a better understanding of the thoughts behind your assessment of risk, you may want to walk through which types of protection you want to use in which scenario.

TIME WALKTHROUGH

Even if you don't have any partners currently, it might help to get into using a calendar regularly to schedule your time and set certain times aside for certain activities. If you're in a couple that's beginning to open up, as aforementioned, it's a good idea to begin to schedule some time apart so that you can get used to the idea of spending more time apart than you do currently, if you don't already.

There is a running joke that one of the most frequently used applications by polyamorous people is Google Calendar and it's most likely because it makes it far easier to work with multiple schedules at once. Even if you are single or you have just one partner, it is still worth scheduling some specific dedicated time to spend away from home or dedicated to a task that's specifically for you.

You may not need every single one of these categories, but it might be worth talking through and seeing if you have each of these categories met.

Do you have time set aside to spend dedicated to yourself? How frequent is this time and why?

. . . .

. . . .

. . . .

Do you have time set aside to spend dedicated to each individual relationship on its own? How frequent is this time and why?

. . . .

. . . .

. . . .

Do you have time set aside to spend dedicated to a dynamic like a triad, quad or else to spend all together? How frequent is this time and why?

. . . .
. . . .
. . . .

Do you have time set aside to spend dedicated to family? How frequent is this time and why?

. . . .
. . . .
. . . .

Do you have time set aside to spend dedicated to children, if you have them? How frequent is this time and why?

. . . .
. . . .
. . . .

Do you have time set aside to spend dedicated to friends? How frequent is this time and why?

. . . .
. . . .
. . . .

What other responsibilities or issues take up your time?

. . . .
. . . .
. . . .

Can anything be done by others to provide you with more time?

. . . .

. . . .

. . . .

What obstacles with time do you face that others may not?

. . . .

. . . .

. . . .

What ways can your partners or others in your life reconcile any struggles you face?

. . . .

. . . .

. . . .

Describe the last time you changed plans. What was your reasoning for it and why?

. . . .

. . . .

. . . .

Describe your thought process for how you prioritize your time.

. . . .

. . . .

. . . .

Are there events or times when you are intentionally not contactable and why?

. . . .

. . . .

. . . .

How do you decide when you are not contactable?

. . . .

. . . .

. . . .

Are there agreements you have within any relationship about how you prioritize your time?

. . . .

. . . .

. . . .

It would be good to work through these alone and then compare answers with your partners, if you have them. As you complete them, you can think about the ways you assume your partners may answer them or what your ideal situation might be when it comes to time management.

SELF-CARE EMERGENCY PROTOCOL

It's best not to wait for a dire situation to happen before taking steps to take care of yourself. Having a protocol that you will use when you begin to experience anxiety or difficult feelings will help you and your partners work through your feelings.

Too many people try to avoid difficult feelings and don't really come up with any protocol for how they might address it or they immediately make rules to have their partner help them manage these feelings while out on a date. There are a lot of ways to manage these feelings without necessarily interrupting a partner while they are out with others.

This is not to say you should never interrupt your partner if they're out with others – consider the previous examples given of your partner being out with family members or children. While you might be experiencing more anxiety and distress than times when your partner is with family members or children, remembering those boundaries can help you make a considered decision.

The following are potential sources of support you can draw upon when you're feeling distressed. Arrange them from whom you are most to least likely to reach out to. You can do this activity on your own or with a partner. Once you have arranged them, go through each section and explain what type of resources you have and why. Once you're done, highlight or underline where you might go in an emergency situation and explain why. You can do this verbally or in a journal.

- Partners

- Friends

- Family members

- Mentors

- Colleagues

- Professionals (e.g. therapist, life coach)

- Social groups/communities

- Helplines

Recognizing what resources you do or don't have and what resources your partners do or don't have can help you understand how they and you manage distress and emergency situations and have more compassion for one another.

What Might You Feel?

∞

Although you're non-monogamous when you decide that that is the style of relationship that you want to have, when you actually put these concepts into practice, you're beginning to call your own bluff. I've personally found that it's particularly easy to believe that you will be fine in words, but the practice is completely different, or it becomes far more difficult than you think.

This chapter will focus on some of the obstacles that you'll likely encounter when it comes to emotions, coping with change and some of the unique challenges that polyamory can bring.

UNEXPECTED BUMPS

Everyone is introduced to non-monogamy in a different way. An easy assumption, and one that I definitely made, was that the more research I did, the more prepared I would be for the 'practice' of non-monogamy. Even though I didn't necessarily begin with a fully realized ideal, I thought that doing the reading would prepare me for a lot more than it actually did.

In some instances, doing the reading made some of the unexpected bumps *worse*, simply because I thought everything could easily be handled by rationalizing my way out of it.

The freedom of non-monogamy

A lot about the philosophy of polyamory and non-monogamy questions some of the more toxic versions of monogamy that society endorses, specifically if you choose forms of non-monogamy that are critical of and seek to reject hierarchy and encourage individual autonomy. Even if you are not open about being non-monogamous or you appear to be monogamous because you only have one partner, deciding to pursue non-monogamy can lead you to challenge some of the assumptions about relationships that are encouraged in monogamy-centric cultures.

My personal discovery of non-monogamy came through the sex-positive community, a community that also was interested in challenging the cultural assumptions around sex that I grew up with. These communities aren't perfect by any means. There were and are a lot of ways that the sex-positive communities I was in failed me as both a person on the asexual spectrum and a sexual assault survivor. But they were my first attempts at calling into question the less helpful ideas that I grew up listening to and absorbing through my culture.

People who practise polyamory or non-monogamy may be more likely to challenge some of the assumptions people make about monogamy and humanity's 'natural' inclination towards it, but that doesn't mean that everyone who practises polyamory is inherently committed to any form of challenge to any power structure. Attempting to get rid of hierarchical structures within society and arguing for polyamory to be included *within* the hierarchy can look like a similar fight, but they are actually very different.

On the outside, for a lot of people, especially if they have no previous experience engaging in any form of protest, social action or challenging any system of power, non-monogamy itself can appear like an inherently more liberating and socially ethical choice. While I have absolutely no doubt that those individuals are speaking truth to their experiences when they say that non-monogamy feels like a more ethical choice for them, their assumption that all the toxic things about monogamy are inherent to the entire practice of monogamy results in the assumption that monogamy itself is unethical or worse.

There are probably many people who go through the experience of encountering a group or practice, learning from that group and practice and then forgetting their own previous ignorance. Unfortunately, this experience sometimes also comes with a phase of looking down on people who were once just as ignorant as you were. But monogamy doesn't inherently have anything to do with being possessive, jealous or even necessarily having a problem with a partner falling in love with someone else.

It's possible to practise monogamy without going through your partner's phone, without keeping tabs on whom they spend their time with, without reacting violently to them flirting with someone else, and I would argue that it's possible to practise monogamy in a way that doesn't assume that romantic relationships are inherently more valuable than any other relationships. Those are all behaviours that are encouraged by the culture around us and by consumer capitalism, which uses our understandable fear of being alone to motivate us into a competition of scarcity and alienates us from other connections.

Non-monogamy can feel freeing because there are many things that you might have to challenge in order to accept the idea as something that you want to even try. If you're the type of person who can't even stand the idea that your partner may find someone else attractive, non-monogamy probably isn't going to be something you want to try. But that doesn't mean non-monogamy is inherently more ethical (which is why I never use the phrase 'ethical non-monogamy'), liberating or even necessarily a better choice for anyone.

The result of this mistake is pretty apparent in a good deal of polyamory communities. Open disdain and mocking of monogamy as a life choice can be tolerated and encouraged in a lot of communities. And while it might be that being on the autistic spectrum means I don't really get these 'jokes', the constant suggestion that being polyam will solve people's romantic problems is a frequent theme. There are also a lot of representations in the media of situations that are very clearly cheating, which are shared to communities as 'accidental polyamory'. Again, it might be my autistic sensibilities making me a bit more of a wet blanket in this instance, but I find these more frustrating than helpful.

At one point, I did also make the assumption that in order to be polyamorous, one had to go through some type of emotional introspection and in order to continue to have 'successful' relationships, one had to be an excellent communicator. I assumed that polyamory involved more 'advanced' skills in relationships than monogamy did. I've now realized that the complexity of any given relationship depends on the people involved. Just like playing a video game 500 times doesn't necessarily mean you've perfected the game mechanics or can play any other game without making any mistakes, the 'success' of any given relationship depends on a lot of uncontrollable factors that you can't account for through your own interpersonal skills alone.

It's important to remember the difference between non-monogamy being a liberating practice for *yourself* and the assumption that non-monogamy is inherently liberating for *everyone*. You may initially feel liberated, and that's fine, but don't let it go to your head and ego.

The wrong ways

There is a lot of discussion within polyamory communities about the actual 'wrong ways' to practise non-monogamy. The aforementioned 'one penis policy' or OPP refers to a situation where, typically, a heterosexual cis man in a relationship with a bisexual cis woman requests or demands that she exclusively dates women, usually cis women. Many people find this discriminatory because the assumption seems to be that the man has no reason to be threatened by his partner dating women and there is also very rarely the recognition that women who have penises and men who have vaginas exist, and that's not even saying anything about where non-binary people are meant to fall in this rule.

While I can't say I'm down with OPP (sorry, couldn't resist), I do think that there are probably a lot of situations where the woman in that relationship is more interested in pursuing relationships with women and therefore might not be that interested in relationships with men. She might agree to this sort of rule because she doesn't intend to seek relationships with men anyway. Likewise, it makes sense to feel less anxiety if your partner is dating people who are, in your mind, so different from you that you don't compare yourself directly to them in the same ways.

I know I have found I felt less anxiety when I had partners dating people who had different gender presentations and identities to me because I had no interest in embodying those presentations so it didn't feel like a comparison. Also, if I knew the partner in question had a different type of anatomy to me, I would then feel like a direct comparison was also more difficult for me to do and, therefore, I would feel less anxious overall. I would probably still advise against this type of hard and fast rule because, as I've mentioned, you can't control your own feelings and in general I think this type of rule is going to be more trouble than it's worth in the end. But, if both parties agree, it's not necessarily completely unethical.

Another commonly criticized practice is the 'veto'. This is where one partner has the power to essentially demand that their partner dump another partner or partners they have. This is different to requesting a return to monogamy or requesting closing the relationship. While I do see vetoes as an inherently unethical practice that could be easily abused by the wrong kind of person, I don't think the desire to want the power of a veto always comes from a malevolent place or even a desire to control a *person*. The criticism of the practice may be valid, but the criticism within polyamory communities towards people who want or try to exercise a veto is often...a little extreme.

Not everyone who desires to have veto power is an evil over-lord. Not everyone who asks their partner to dump someone else is doing so in an attempt to be controlling or abusive. I've seen vetoes used as desperate measures by people who felt like it was the only way to keep their relationship from slipping out of their fingers. And in fairness to those people, if one of the main problems is someone neglecting one relationship because they're so invested in another, a veto technically *does* address that problem – but if your partner is not committed to you, no veto can fix that.

I have yet to see a situation in which one person wanted a veto where there weren't some deeper issues that the veto wouldn't really solve. You can't force a partner to be more atten-tive, to communicate, to value you, to stop dating someone who is hurting them or to do anything really, and even if you can force them to dump someone else, that's typically not really the point. Vetoes are also horrible for the people who are getting dumped, especially if they had no idea that someone had veto power over their relationship. If you plan on exercising a veto, it's always best to advise your other partners that one partner does have this power.

Another frequently criticized practice is 'unicorn hunters', as defined in the Glossary. While I can totally understand why this practice has broken hearts and garnered a negative reputation in the community, I have also heard from people who prefer engaging with couples and have never had this experience.

I think sometimes the community can be too harsh on people who are brand new to polyamory and decide to go about it in this way out of ignorance or fear. It makes sense that people new to polyamory would try what they consider to be the 'safest' way to experience a form of non-monogamy without understanding what it must be like for the 'third' person. That's not to excuse people who hurt others in their ignorance, but I don't think the assumption that people are trying to use and abuse someone if they seem to tick all the unicorn hunting boxes is correct. If you have considered this type of approach to non-monogamy, I would definitely urge you to date as individuals simply because the task of dating a couple is more daunting for a lot of people than it is exciting.

And finally, another frequently criticized practice is 'don't ask, don't tell', or DADT. Based on the US government approach to queer people in the military, DADT is usually where one person in a couple gives the other permission to do what they'd like on a certain date or dates with whomever but doesn't want to be told about it and wants to continue the appearance of being a monogamous couple on the outside to friends and family. I absolutely understand why many people would see this practice as unethical, but at the same time, I think if this situation works for both people and they both consent to it, then it isn't inherently unethical.

What I feel is unethical is not disclosing to any individuals you have dates or anything else with that you have this setup. It's important that if you are going to clearly prioritize one of your partners and keep the rest secret that you at least give people the chance to consent to that from the outset. Some people don't mind or might even be super-interested in dating or sleeping with someone in that kind of setup and others would become unhappy with it over time or would never want to be involved. All opinions about how to be involved with someone in a DADT relationship are valid approaches and feelings. As long as expectations are clear on both sides, I think it can be a rational choice for some people that doesn't have to break hearts.

While vetoes, unicorn hunting, DADT or OPPs aren't necessarily rules directly from monogamy, the concept of one partner having a preference over others is arguably a hangover from the toxic aspect of monogamy which encourages people to value one romantic relationship over all other types of relationships. These tend to be one of the only types of hangovers people want to address, but there are other aspects I've witnessed within polyamory communities that go unchallenged.

This is absolutely not a universal rule. As I've mentioned before, polyamory communities in my experience are postcode lotteries at times – meaning that you may end up in a situation where you live in an area with a very supportive community that's understanding or even has a lot of racial, gender, life experience and other diversities...or you might not. But in my experience, in a lot of polyamory communities a good deal of the heavy lifting and work is often placed on the shoulders of women. This means organizing work, childcare, as well as the harder aspects of creating and sustaining a community. Men tend to be individually famous and have personal celebrity while a lot of women are working in the background to make things actually happen.

And in many communities, the women who tend to be the centre of organizing and volunteering tend to be those women who have the free time and emotional energy to do so – which tends to be white and wealthier women. Again, I'm not saying all communities are like this, but I have witnessed a good many that are and found it extremely odd considering how polyamory is meant to challenge the status quo – then why does it seem like a lot of the hard and unwanted work tends to fall on women? Perhaps it's because I'm non-binary and will quite often be placed into a segregated role against my will that I've noticed the disparity in the level of work and the mismatch of representation.

It's important for women going into polyamorous communities to be aware of the space they occupy as well as the assumptions that they have when organizing. While I don't necessarily see it as a problem that women want to devote voluntary and free time to a polyamory community, the issue is that whenever something must be done unpaid or in free time, you will automatically limit the pool of people who have the energy, time or money to give. This inherently affects the diversity of the community and the people who make decisions and, whenever women of colour are involved, they may be expected to do the additional labour of providing the rest of the group with anti-racist education or deal with the lack of perspective offered by the community quietly.

If you have the free time to organize a polyamory event, then you have the free time to educate yourself and not be shocked when a Black or Brown person tells you that they have experienced racism in the polyamory community. Likewise, understand that if a person tells you they have experienced any marginalization or people ignoring or sidelining their needs, listen and respect that experience. Organizing events, even when you do have the free time and energy, can be difficult and you won't necessarily get everything right all the time.

The difficulty of organizing that many face sometimes also stems from people's inability or unwillingness to ask for help when they need it and the fact that women often grow up expecting to labour for love. It's always important, if you feel powerless, to understand that you usually have more power than you give yourself credit for. There is really no good reason why the division of labour exists in so many polyamory communities in such an unequal way. And those men who would consider themselves allies need to take a strong role in doing the labour, not just the leadership, within communities.

But maybe you have a queerer community where the division of labour isn't so feminized or made up mainly of those with the privilege of time, economy and energy to devote themselves to running community events. I certainly hope that is the case! But just be aware when approaching your communities of this imbalance of labour. Because it's also something I quite often see mirrored in relationships as well in both my personal experience and in the advice I've given. I don't think I've received a single letter from a man trying to ask me how to build a better relationship with a metamour but multiple letters from women whose male partners left it up to the women to decide to work it out instead of establishing their own boundaries and taking ownership of them.

Giving permission

Non-monogamy isn't given to us in any real cultural script, though people are aware that 'open relationships' do exist. Again, I wouldn't be surprised if most people believed 'open relationships don't work'. It makes sense that people would feel understandably anxious when they try non-monogamy for the first time. And in that anxiety what a lot of people either want to give to their partners or receive from their partners is reassurance.

I've already written about why reassurance can be a double-edged sword, but one of the first mistakes people make is asking for reassurance by way of requesting permission for certain things. If you are with someone who is especially anxious of being rejected, getting in 'trouble', or who has a lot of specific anxieties around upsetting you, then it can become incredibly difficult learning how to tell the difference between reaffirming your consent to non-monogamy and giving 'permission'.

Giving permission usually manifests in the form of having your partner ask you 'Is it okay if I sleep with X?' or even making a rule that you have to meet or 'discuss' people before they become your partner. The issue with permission is that, while it may provide temporary relief to the person asking for it, what it can often feel like for the person giving it is, 'You have one chance to be unhappy about this and that's it'. Even if you don't have the type of relationship where your partner wouldn't be sympathetic to you being upset, you can still feel like giving permission is almost like promising you won't freak out. Or potentially you feel comforted by giving permission because you don't trust yourself to cope with the news otherwise without freaking out.

For someone who is worried about being blamed for something going wrong, in the same way people worry about being accused of cheating, getting permission is your get out of jail free card and a way of proving that you did everything that you can do and therefore are not responsible for the emotions your partner has – or at least maybe you attack yourself less if you get permission first if your partner becomes upset later.

While I feel like I have a good understanding of what will and won't upset me, I absolutely categorically refuse to give 'permission' for individual partners, individual situations or anything which basically means I'm expected to predict what my emotions might be like, and I have had partners who have constantly tried to put me in a position of giving permission to soothe their *own* anxiety about a situation. While it may seem like no big deal to give permission or might even be comforting to some, there are lots of ways this can manifest as more problems later.

If your problem tends to be that your partner doesn't check in with you or establish any regular connection with you, then asking for permission can feel like that type of communication. In one relationship I had, during the visit of what was supposed to be 'just a friend', I had a partner consistently come and spend time with me in a way that he had never done before. During the visit, I wasn't actually that bothered, because I was getting attention that I had never got before. But later on when I realized that this attention was temporary and just for the duration of the visit, it didn't end up solving problems, just making them worse.

In other situations, I have been expected to give permission for my partner to sleep with someone whom I don't particularly like or care for. I have and do consent to non-monogamy and I don't believe it's my place to control the decision of whom my partners sleep with. But I can't promise to be happy and ecstatic over their every choice. I can't promise that I won't have any feelings if they choose someone who has treated me poorly. While I'm unlikely to dump them purely for deciding to sleep with someone who once wronged me, I'm also not likely going to want a life where I share a lot of time and personal space with that person.

A similar situation to this often arises when monogamous people have partners who have friends or family they don't like, except very rarely do we expect people in that case to give permission to hang out with those people. We might feel like we have to negotiate shared spaces if someone comes to visit, but the issue of permission doesn't really arise – or shouldn't if the relationship is healthy. We also don't expect that our partners would break up with us because of our friends or family, even though that can and does happen when situations get dire.

You have to operate with an understanding in your partnership, if you have both agreed to be non-monogamous, that you trust one another. If you have a discussion about how you want to practise polyamory then you should have an understanding of the relationships that you may want to have with your partner's partners or metamours, which should help manage your anxiety around what might be expected in terms of how you might be interacting with your metamours. At the end of the day, your partner is the hinge between you two and you have to have faith that your partner will be able to manage the problems that come up in that relationship without it having to be about blame or without it being your responsibility to manage.

Likewise, if you are a person who finds yourself wanting to ask if your partner is 'okay' with certain partners or certain things happening with certain partners, doing some work with a polyamory-friendly therapist on your own anxiety might help you avoid needing that specific type of reassurance. Your partner cannot always guarantee that they won't have an emotional reaction to someone you choose to date or even have a crush on. You have to be able to trust that they are able to manage their emotions and, if they feel like they need your help, that they will come to you. You can still have regular check-ins and discussions to address problems as and when they may arise, but understand that asking for 'permission' in this way can often cause more problems in the long run. There isn't anything that permission solves that wouldn't be solved by communication and trust on both sides.

Self-attack and isolation

One of the most difficult things I found myself experiencing in non-monogamy was understanding when to trust myself and when to voice my concerns. Specifically, when I was starting out in non-monogamy, I had a lot of experiences I would not have had if I trusted my gut and intuition. The problem with a lot of the advice I read when I was beginning to have my first non-monogamous relationships was that so much of what I read encouraged me to always question my emotions.

Perhaps for someone who doesn't have anxiety or who doesn't struggle with mental health issues, the concept of questioning your feelings is novel. Someone who has anxiety spends all their time second, third and fourth guessing themselves, so co-signing this as a concept or way to approach relationships is almost like shooting oneself in the foot. For myself, I never trusted any assumption I made and also assumed that any negative feeling I had was some type of inherent jealousy I had picked up from a monogamous culture – even though some of the negative feelings I had were justified.

Getting caught in a wheel of feeling bad for feeling bad was a frequent trap I would find myself in within non-monogamy. I tried so hard to prevent myself from being this caricature of a jealous, controlling partner, especially since I had gone through so much with controlling people. I knew what it was like for someone to watch my every move, waiting for me to mess up. Having gone through difficult relationships where I was mistreated or abused, my biggest fear was to become one of those people.

I desperately wanted to be a good example, to take to polyamory like a fish to water and prove my own emotional intelligence to my partners. I felt like it wasn't impossible for me to do, especially since I hadn't had many monogamous relationships and wasn't really wedded to the idea in its entirety. Putting so much pressure on myself made it more difficult when I did actually begin to have problems. I had learned so much about what *not to do* that I realized when I started delving into situations where I might be jealous that I had no idea what *to do* instead.

It was super easy for me to get into a pit where everything

that went wrong was inherently my fault and a lot of common narratives in polyamory advice only supported that. After all, my emotions were my responsibility to manage, right? And if I kept having problems then the common denominator in all those problems was myself, right? It never once occurred to me that attacking myself might be the source of a lot of different problems I was having in my life. And even now, I struggle not to slip into self-attack when something goes wrong.

Polyamory advice often encourages you to handle all your problems on your own. Telling a partner that you're not feeling great about something is never news that you want to deliver. That, combined with the fact that usually needing to 'talk' in a monogamous relationship is a dubious sign, can mean you easily get stuck in a trap where you feel even more isolated, especially if you have no one else in your life you can talk to about non-monogamy.

Not every non-monogamous person has a family or friendship network that is open to non-monogamy and, even if they are, they may not feel they have the skillset to provide advice, or their advice may be seriously unhelpful (e.g. don't be non-monogamous then). And even some therapists have little experience in non-monogamy or have a prejudice against it, especially if the person practising it is more likely to be shamed for engaging in any forms of sexuality.

While I do think it's helpful for people to find a polyamory friendly therapist to talk to about any issues you might be processing, I also think it's important for people to avoid putting themselves into a position of self-attack isolation. Specifically, therapists can help you find a balance between letting your partner know about your feelings and working through them together and turning your partner into a therapist. Relying on your partner as you would a therapist puts a huge burden on them, but this doesn't mean that every single emotion you have that isn't happiness should be hidden.

You won't always get this balance perfect and, for me especially, what helped me when I was trying to work out this balance was having a partner who understood that I was passive aggressive when I was afraid and didn't know how to communicate my needs. I still struggle with figuring out when to have a confrontation and when a confrontation is even necessary or understanding that stating my needs doesn't have to be a confrontation. I've been able to figure out how to get out of that cycle of self-attack and isolating myself, but it takes work not to put myself back into that spiral.

Sometimes when you have a relationship that rarely has problems, that means you won't get the chance to actively deal with these issues all the time, which means it may be a little bit more time before you make improvements in a way that you notice. Don't get discouraged by that. One of the things that is most helpful to learn to get yourself out of a cycle of self-attack is self-compassion. Beating yourself up for having feelings doesn't make those feelings go away, it just creates new feelings and new difficulties.

Having compassion for your feelings will be incredibly difficult at first, especially if you've been raised with the idea that having compassion for yourself is weakness and your survival instincts tell you that showing weakness will result in some type of attack towards you. It is a muscle that you have to continue to engage in order to keep strong, so try to keep that in mind as you start to have your first experiences.

METAMOURS AND BOUNDARIES

Negotiating the boundaries you have with metamours is another tricky aspect of polyamory that will largely depend on how you envision your life and how flexible that picture can be. While you may frequently hear 'there is no one right way to do polyamory', the implicit suggestion – through concepts like 'compersion' and the way jealousy is derided – is that the ideal way is one where you embrace metamours as friends.

Not everyone is going to have the same boundaries and feelings towards metamours and there are lots of challenges that might arise when it comes to metamours that you may not have much experience with – or at least think you don't – if you're new to non-monogamy.

'Success' in polyamory

Across the spectrum of relationship types, we tend to assume that a 'successful' relationship is one that lasts until someone in the relationship doesn't make it out alive. To a certain extent, this makes sense. Breakups, even ones that are mutually decided upon, aren't usually fun experiences. Usually losing relationships, regardless of what type, is painful and it makes sense to want to avoid painful experiences. But a stagnant and unfulfilling relationship you feel like you can't escape is also a different type of pain that's difficult to ignore.

Non-monogamy can add an extra pressure in that proving that you are 'good at polyamory' often means having a lot of long-term relationships and breaking up can feel like it's not just losing a relationship, but a sign that you aren't good at polyamory. This pressure could contribute towards people staying in polyamorous relationships longer than they might if it were a monogamous relationship or feeling especially ashamed when a breakup does happen.

Furthermore, even though there is 'no one right way to do polyamory' as mentioned previously, the concept of compersion creates a suggested preference, which is one where you get along with all your partner's partners at the very least. Even without this pressure, we will often find ourselves wanting to get along with our metamours and become friends with them in the same way that in monogamous relationships we want our partner's family or friends to like us. The difference when it comes to metamours is that the stakes feel slightly higher, perhaps even higher than a partner's family member disliking you. If you are dating someone who is also interested in another partner you have, that can further add to the pressure of you wanting to make sure you make a good impression, so you don't somehow 'ruin it' for others.

For many people, family relationships aren't something easily ruined. My family relationships have not stood the test of time and that has contributed towards me putting pressure on myself to befriend metamours. Part of me has blamed myself for 'ruining' my family and thus believing I have the power to 'ruin' my partner's relationships when it just isn't as simple as that. Responding to that fear by pushing myself to befriend metamours I wouldn't be friends with in normal circumstances did not lead me to a good place.

But there is only so much you can control as an individual. Someone who has the best communication skills and excellent boundaries cannot make up for someone else who doesn't. And in some cases, people can be decent, nice and wonderful, but still incompatible. Defining 'success' just as being in a relationship for a long time doesn't work for monogamy and it doesn't work for non-monogamy for a lot of reasons. Equally assuming that not getting along with or caring for a metamour means failure puts an unfair burden on yourself to make a friendship where you normally wouldn't.

If you feel self-conscious because of a breakup or feel a pressure to stay in a relationship to prove how 'good' you are at non-monogamy or are forcing yourself to be closer to a metamour than you normally would, reconsider that assumption and thought process. Focus less on what other people might consider success and ask yourself what lies behind what you consider success.

Relationship by force

If you feel pressure to get along with your metamours applied by yourself, your surrounding community, your partner or any combination of these, you might end up in a lot of difficult situations. My feelings about my relationships to metamours have changed throughout my experiences. Initially, after being used to cheat, it was important to me to meet my metamours so that I was sure I wasn't being used to cheat. Also, my experience of being blamed by a metamour made me even more anxious about 'ruining it'.

Metamours can also put you in situations where you feel like you're forced to discuss what's going on in you and your partner's relationship in front of them. I've had positive relationships with metamours, but as yet none of them have become my best friends because just dating the same person isn't necessarily enough to create a friendship. While we have had a fair bit in common because partners I have had have tended to be interested in similar people, I feel like there is an underlying pressure I still put on myself, even though I know better, to get things 'right' in a way that will always prevent me from being really close to any metamour.

For a short period of time, I attempted to force myself into a friendship with a metamour and the result of that was a specific and noticeable increase in my anxiety and forced conversations that I didn't enjoy or benefit from. For some people, this may not be an issue. When I consider the other aspects of life where I feel I'm forced to have a relationship based on a small commonality, like working in the same environment, I have an equal amount of frustration. That's not to say I can't make friends with people at work, but, again, the stakes are different when I cannot just choose to simply disengage with a person.

There was a lot in my life growing up, including going by a different name at home and at school, facing a large amount of bullying and trying to understand my own bisexual identity, which caused me to have a different approach to identity. Not to mention, a lot of autistic people deal with what's called 'masking' where we often have to learn and recreate behaviours that we witness non-autistic people doing in order to be socially accepted.

Because of that, I've been quite used to keeping my guard up and keeping a firm barrier between the public and the private. This continues into the workplace for me now, even though I feel I'm less likely to be cornered in a bathroom by a group of bullies. In many cases, it's better to keep work relationships as professional as possible. For some people, this has never been an issue; forming casual relationships with people in workplaces, school and metamours has never been a problem for them and they don't have a separation between the public and the private in the same way I do.

If that's the case and having a casual friendship with a metamour doesn't cause your hair to stand on end, then that's great. I'm definitely far more relaxed about metamours now than I used to be and now only feel more anxious if I have a partner who is anxious about me becoming anxious. For some people, bringing their metamour around their partner or having shared events where they interact makes *them* so anxious that it defeats the purpose.

The point is that, regardless of what side of the situation you're on, if you're so anxious that the relationship becomes difficult, don't force yourself into it because you feel you have something to prove to yourself, the community or to anyone else. Forcing myself into situations where I was socially interacting with a metamour made me uncomfortable and short-tempered. It wasn't worth it and it didn't really do anything helpful for me. You're not a failure if you don't want to meet or engage with any metamours and it isn't a DADT relationship just because you're not besties with your metamours.

Opportunism

Another obstacle that may cause difficulty when trying to associate with metamours may be when it seems that your partner has been motivated to try polyamory because of an opportunity to be with someone else. And if the partner is unfamiliar with polyamory or hasn't tried it before (though people who have tried polyamory before could also make this mistake) they might not have been honest about the potentiality of the opportunity from the beginning.

It can be particularly hard not to displace the frustration of such a massive change onto a metamour. Having to face the potentiality of losing your partner, changing your relationship style, having to counteract all the monogamy-centric information you've absorbed all of your life and develop a positive relationship with the person who you feel has 'caused' this cataclysmic change in your life can be incredibly difficult for even a confident and self-assured person to manage. It's a lot of change and feels very sudden. I would liken it to the feeling of resentment and anger that some children have when they learn they have a new sibling on the way.

That's not to say these feelings are childish, but that it might be difficult for you, especially in a time when you're trying to re-establish trust and love with your partner in a different style of relationship, not to *also* hold some frustration and anger with them for the cost of the opportunity they wanted to take advantage of. It might feel hard to not feel cheated and lied to, even if your partner never intended for that to happen. It can be hard not to feel left behind or ignored, especially if your partner is brimming with new relationship energy and it feels like you've been left to pick up the pieces.

The important thing to remember when you're on this side of the exchange is that introducing the subject of polyamory into a monogamous relationship can absolutely be downright dangerous. Given the messages that societies often teach about monogamy, it makes sense that many may often react badly to the thought that their partner desires or wants someone other than them. It might be so painful to acknowledge that it threatens the fabric of the relationship.

Some people may feel an inclination towards polyamory but have no real idea that it's what they want until they see and know another person whom they want to have a relationship with. They may not feel sure about reaching out and having that discussion with their partner until there is a tangible chance of another partner they could potentially have, which makes it worth the risk to ask about it. They may have gone back and forth while their feelings for this other person have bubbled up. Not everyone can be self-aware enough to grasp the point when they begin to develop feelings for someone and may not really know until it's more or less 'too late'.

I've received many letters from people who have experienced a lot of pressure from their partner to open up because an opportunity has presented itself for them to enter into a relationship with another person. The pressure makes a difficult situation more difficult and I can often see it from the perspective of both sides. On the one hand, I can understand the freedom in finally admitting to yourself that this is what you want and the excitement of another potential relationship on your doorstep. So many people have rushed into relationships in monogamy so we're liable to do that when it comes to polyamory. Chemistry can be a difficult thing to ignore or deny.

On the other hand, for someone who has gone from monogamy and the illusion of safety it provides to suddenly having to try a new relationship style that they may have never heard of or only heard bad things about and then also have a partner who seems extremely keen to *not* be with you...this change can feel so sudden it causes emotional whiplash. Additional pressure makes an already difficult situation that much more difficult.

Unless someone involved has a terminal illness, there is often no reason to rush things. If you find yourself in a situation where you are interested in someone and feel like you want your partner's official and complete seal of approval of polyamory *before* you even approach the discussion of polyamory with someone you've been flirting with...you're really not setting yourself up well in either situation. A lot of people seem to be under the impression that they will have complete control over their partner's perception or willingness to try polyamory if they introduce the idea well enough.

While it's true that if you introduce the concept of trying a new restaurant to your partner by comparing the type of food the restaurant serves to something disgusting, you may influence your partner not to want to try it, at the end of the day your partner will either like the food or won't. Introducing polyamory to your partner *without* being honest about having feelings for someone else runs the risk that they will understandably feel bad and I have absolutely seen people crash the polyamory cart into the aisle of their relationship and run off with the person they wanted to sleep with and ignore the mess they've created. It's not always easy to introduce the concept to your partner, but the problem often isn't with whether polyamory is something someone can do but whether or not their partner is willing to be patient, kind and caring.

Not to mention, you could very well introduce the concept of polyamory to your partner, which will, especially if they haven't heard of or don't have interest in it, cause some stress, only to find out the person you've been flirting with is either not interested in polyamory or, worse, has a thing for helping people cheat and finds the idea of your partner knowing about you being with someone else and being okay with it less fun. If someone who is interested in you knows you as monogamous and is openly flirting with you, this may not be the polyamory ideal you think it is and that is always worth considering.

Practical honesty with both parties and honesty with yourself is probably best advised. I often encourage people, if they seriously think they want polyamory, to accept that this could mean the end of their monogamous relationship and also to introduce the concept of polyamory to a partner by watching something with a polyamorous character or finding an article on polyamory and starting a discussion about it.

Another way to begin a discussion is by talking about the

concept of the 'free pass' within monogamy, which is where you name a celebrity you would have a 'free pass' to sleep with if the situation ever arose. Or there are a few celebrities who have had public discussions about them having open relationships (Will Smith and Jada Pinkett-Smith are a frequent example) you can bring up. Someone's reaction to those discussion topics might give you the understanding you need about their willingness to try or be receptive to polyamory.

If you get a positive response from either party you're interested in, it's worth considering finding a polyamory-friendly couples therapist or making sure your therapist is also receptive to the concept, if that is accessible to you. It's important for you to understand how much of a hard limit polyamory is for you. Some people would be happy to be in either relationship style, but understand that once the cat is out of the proverbial bag, it will be out. Even if you claim you will be okay with monogamy, your partner may continue to be worried that they are preventing you from a life you secretly want.

Don't expect your partner to welcome the topic completely and don't put pressure on them to be perfectly okay with everything before you approach the other person. Be honest with the other person that you're at the beginning of this journey and going through a lot. People tend to be afraid of being fully honest with newer partners and want everything to happen without any bumps, but I think often pretending to be okay ends up causing a lot more difficulties. While it may seem more fun and enjoyable to begin polyamory with two partners, I do think, especially if everyone in the situation is new to polyamory, this presents a particularly difficult challenge for the hinge, or the person in the middle, to try and keep everything balanced.

If you're on the opposite side of the situation, it's important to remember that your brain might find it easier to blame the new metamour for all the shifts and difficulties in the relationship instead of focusing on the issue you actually have with your partner. That's not to say a metamour, especially one new to polyamory, can't cause problems. Cowboying, Cowgirling or Cowpoking can be a thing – which is where a person enters into a relationship with someone who is polyamorous with the express intention of stealing them from the other person.

While a metamour can absolutely make things more difficult, it does take two to tango, so to say. If you have a metamour who is disparaging you verbally for example in front of your partner and your partner does nothing about it or doesn't seem to have a problem with it, while it's true that your metamour is being a jerk, the bigger issue is that your partner doesn't seem to have a problem with you being insulted and isn't trying to stop that from happening.

Understand that, even if it feels opportunistic, this can happen to the most honest of us. It's not necessarily malice if your partner was unsure about whether to bring up polyamory until they had an opportunity to date someone else. Make sure that you do the exploration needed and outlined at the beginning of this book to see if polyamory is meant for you and identify what your needs are. If you have a partner who refuses to have these basic exploratory discussions with you and looks like they were just waiting for a green light before abandoning you, that is something they need to be responsible for and stop doing even if they don't realize they are doing it.

Taking advantage of an opportunity is understandable, but that doesn't mean pressuring a partner. Taking steps to understand the receptiveness to polyamory of the people you're interested in, respecting that the decision to change your relationship style will be stressful (especially if it wasn't your idea and you've had no familiarity with it) and being willing to be there for your partner and have those discussions without getting swept up in new relationship energy are all important. And if you are experiencing a huge amount of neglect from your partner after they asked you to try polyamory, then it's worth considering whether it's them that's not cut out for having multiple partners rather than yourself.

Again, polyamory is not monogamy with an upgrade that includes cheating with permission. It's a different way of doing things that might be more difficult for a lot of people who have been raised in monogamy-centric cultures and who have no blueprint to follow. Even for people who have cheated before and even for people who have a huge interest in non-monogamy, it can be stressful when you move from theory to practice.

Negotiation and blaming

Another aspect that can be difficult is if your partner in common or the 'hinge' is putting the responsibility for negotiating everything on you or your metamours instead of taking responsibility for it themselves. It can be easy to blame your metamour for being unreasonable or demanding too much time for themselves and I have received a lot of letters from people seeking to have a better relationship with their metamour and believing it's their responsibility to manage.

Typically, I think all people involved having a stronger understanding of what they personally want to get out of polyamory can help avoid a lot of stress. Agreements in a relationship about responsibility and time have to be just that, agreements. At times I've witnessed people deciding to blame their metamour for what is actually their partner's choice of how they spend their time. Particularly this tends to happen to people who have a partnership that was monogamous before they opened the relationship, or those who have a domestic or primary or married partner and end up telling their other partners that they can't call, meet up or keep time commitments because of the feelings of their other partner.

Of course, some people do attempt to control their partners in ways which are abusive, but not all boundary-setting is abusive. If your partner says they don't want you to have phone calls with others within the house you share, and you agree to it, you need to honour the agreement. You can also choose not to agree or to renegotiate it.

I understand this can be tricky, especially if you are making concessions for a partner who is struggling to cope with polyamory and isn't sure it's something they want. Also, if you're living together and you can't just leave, it might put you in a really difficult situation. But you do have to own that you are making a choice that, even if it's not intentional, it will feel like you're prioritizing one partner's comfort over yours and that of your other partner. Blaming your partner for that isn't really fair.

Equally, if you have a partner who is not giving you what you need and, when you ask for it, blames their partner, avoid trying to hold your metamour accountable for that and hold *your partner* accountable for it instead. That can be incredibly difficult because, just like I mentioned in the Opportunism section, it's easier for you to displace anger and frustration onto someone you don't know or even perhaps someone you do know and don't feel great about. It's easier to hold them accountable, especially if you have a partner who does feel powerless.

When I had the experience of my partner giving a metamour something I wanted right in front of me, I broke down and had to retreat to a friend's house to recuperate. This was the last straw in a series of problems that I was trying to convince myself that we didn't have. I was beyond angry and, to make it worse, my metamour wanted me to come back to the house and have a discussion with both of them – even though I knew even then that the issue was specifically with my partner and our relationship and not with my metamour. This wasn't something talking with my metamour could solve.

Of course, I still experienced resentment and frustration towards her because of the way she decided to handle that situation. And when my partner asked if it was okay if they could go and spend the night with this metamour, I was honest that I didn't feel good about it. We were working on a permission basis, which wasn't helpful on top of everything. I had been asked for my permission and I'd given it, not realizing how painful it would be to witness or anticipate my feelings and now I wasn't okay with it so...we felt at a stalemate. Even though I was in a difficult situation, I recognized that the metamour wasn't the issue, it was what was going on with us. But I can't lie – witnessing them getting what I had always wanted did sour the beginning of what friendship they tried to have with me.

I won't pretend it isn't difficult to try and manage the needs and wants of two or more people. It is difficult. But that's why trying your best to have a good understanding of your own needs as an individual as well as what you want within polyamory so you know how to balance your own needs with everyone else's is paramount. If you have no particular preference or aren't able to set down boundaries, then it can become easy for you to adjust them to one particular person and then struggle when you have two people with conflicting boundaries and feelings.

I also acknowledge there may be situations where you are agreeing to your partner's boundaries, but they are not the boundaries that you would put down and so you can feel like having to follow them *is* their fault, in some ways. If the choice is between agreeing to your partner's boundaries and losing them, you can feel like you had no other choice. And, as aforementioned, you might be in an economic situation where leaving is not an option that's easy or even remotely feasible for you. I think it's possible to be honest about boundaries you have agreed to without scapegoating one partner to another.

Getting the balance right is difficult, but it's important to make sure that you and your partners are owning your choices where possible and not allowing other partners to take the fall.

COMPARISON AND COMPERSION

The most frequent feeling people have when their partner asks them to consider polyamory is a sadness that they are not 'enough' for their partner. We're encouraged by consumer capitalism to compare ourselves to others constantly and to consume the right things so that we can effectively compete with one another. Constantly we are sold a warped 'survival of the fittest' narrative where we think that, as we've discussed before, finding a partner is some type of triathlon that you complete to receive your reward.

Even though polyamory does have lots of benefits that can fight against these messages, comparisons can sometimes become a real obstacle for a lot of people in a variety of ways – except where comparing yourself to other partners might make a lot of sense.

Competition and comparison

One of the most common occurrences when an existing monogamous couple 'open up' is that one partner has an easier time finding partners than the other for whatever reason. Typically, if the couple are two heterosexual cis people, women tend to find it easier to find partners for a lot of reasons including getting more attention online (which isn't always a benefit), being approached more often, and quite often men interested in her may suspect she could be cheating but don't care, whereas men tend to not be trusted by single women when they claim to be polyamorous.

It is understandable to be upset that you are not getting any potential dates and a partner is. In some cases, one partner could have really pushed for the other to try non-monogamy and the other partner ends up taking to it well and finding lots of partners, which leaves a special kind of frustration for the other, but this is unfortunately something that can't really be helped. I would encourage people not to assume that more messages on dating websites or more attention necessarily equates to more quality partnerships. Oftentimes having to wade through a wave of initial messages to find someone who is open to polyamory and is compatible with you is overwhelming and difficult. There are a lot of people willing to try polyamory but, depending on your location, not a lot of people have really thought about how their life would be different if they were polyam and it can be extremely daunting to feel like you have to find your way through that.

Many people feel at the outset that even the suggestion of polyamory means they aren't 'good enough' for their partner. And while for most people it may not be as simple as that, if the relationship opened due to an inherent incompatibility between two people, it can be quite difficult not to feel like you're not 'good enough'. Especially if you are a person with a history of comparing yourself to your peers or siblings, comparing yourself to other partners or focusing on what other partners have that you do not can be a pretty natural route for your brain to take.

The polyamory advice that I received when I personally encountered this problem was to remember that I was a unique and wonderful individual and that my partner had their own special reasons for choosing me that no one else could compare to. And while this sounded great on paper, the practice of it felt completely different. I had struggled with low self-worth most of my life and was never really taught to value myself.

The message I personally received growing up was that my worth as a person was inherently connected to how useful I could be or how little trouble I caused anyone. I couldn't see the inherent worth of myself so imagining that a partner could see that was very difficult for me. Originally the advice seemed logical and possible, but when it was time to execute it, my brain just wasn't used to the idea that I had enough worth to keep someone around without being useful and quiet.

Accepting that there was only so much I could control about whether or not my partner stayed with me or valued me helped a lot in releasing that desire to compare myself with others. I found it extremely difficult to engage in positive self-talk initially because it felt fake and awkward. Instead, I shot for neutrality, which was a lot easier to aim for. Making a rule that I could not insult myself or call myself a name instead of trying to push myself to sell all the positive aspects of me was extremely help-ful. Not to mention, defining my personal worth in comparison to what I could offer to another felt like a continuation of the same problems I'd always had – defining my worth by my usefulness to others.

Ultimately there's not a magical solution for fixing a tendency to compare yourself to others and it might be even more confusing when sometimes the comparisons are apt. The rule I try to apply when making comparisons is about whether it is about my partner or about my metamour. If I compare myself to a metamour who cooks better than me, that's less about my partner and their behaviour and more about my metamour, which isn't really something that should impact the relationship between my partner and me. Whereas, if I notice my partner cooks for my metamour but never offers to do so for me, that is less about their relationship and more about our own and that comparison is fairly apt.

Even with the first comparison, it's worth asking how you know your metamour cooks better? Is it because your partner *makes* the comparison through comments? In that case, is that actually about your metamour's behaviour or is that about the fact that your partner is drawing comparisons that criticize you and make you feel like you are not good enough? Really examine whether the comparisons you're making are things you can change or signs of the issues you're having with your own relationship.

While everyone has different relationships with different people, it's okay to want your partner to give you something within your relationship, especially if you see them giving it to another person and you previously believed they just didn't give those things. Be wary of attempting to watch the relationships your partners have even for these comparisons, because ideally you will already have thought about what you needed within your relationship so you should both have a good understanding of that.

Feeling compersion

We've already discussed how the concept of 'compersion' – intended to be the opposite of jealousy – creates a type of ideal, even when we say there is no one right way to do polyamory. It's possible that there are a lot of people who feel no pressure to have 'compersion' whatsoever, but I know that this was the type of ideal that I want to achieve and felt pressure to achieve it so I could prove how much I could 'handle' polyamory.

For me, not feeling 'compersion' immediately became some type of warning sign, let alone if I felt nervous or unhappy or about my partner being with someone else. Putting my reactions and feelings under a microscope made me feel like I was a walking time-bomb. I was always waiting to see whether I would explode and holding my breath to feel the rush of 'compersion' and feeling like something was wrong when it never came.

Feeling neutral about partners dating others felt like a problem initially that I had to repair by being friends with my metamours or trying to challenge my own thoughts about myself. I assumed it was a huge problem that had to be fixed instead of really examining other relationships in my life. But then I thought about it and realized I wasn't necessarily overjoyed or felt 'compersion' for anybody else, like friends or family. Obviously, I'm glad if a friend finds someone new and they feel excited about that, but I don't necessarily feel overjoyed about it. I'm glad that they're happy but that's pretty much the long and the short of it.

It's possible to struggle with self-worth and self-esteem while also feeling neutral about the people or the situations your partner has when it comes to their personal love life. Just because you don't find boundless joy or second-hand excitement because your partner had a one-night stand, has a new crush or started a new relationship is not an indication or a reflection of poor self-esteem, nor does it mean you're not cut out for polyamory. If you're normally overjoyed and excited and you suddenly find yourself neutral, that might be worth examining, but just feeling neutral is not an actual problem or a bad sign.

Most of my desire to feel compersion came from a fear of jealousy. The assumption I had was that if I felt an overwhelming amount of joy, I wouldn't have any room to feel jealousy. Compersion was meant to be my anchor so that when I had feelings of inadequacy when compared to other partners, I could bring myself back to my happiness for my partner. So not having it immediately there was worrying in and of itself. Jealousy definitely felt like something that I connected with a lot of shame. Being jealous as a polyamorous person was a failure, so I was terrified of that prospect.

If compersion isn't really something you feel, that isn't abnormal and it isn't a sign of a deeper problem. When reading through a lot of beginner polyamory advice, you may end up feeling similarly to me in that you're putting a lot of pressure on yourself to experience this feeling or feeling like neutrality means something is wrong. Just keep in mind that different people are different and just because you don't feel it doesn't necessarily mean you're jealous or there's something wrong with you.

Being an emotional gladiator

For some people, they know for sure or quickly if polyamory is for them or they feel confident about trying it. That's not to say that those people will definitely end up feeling the same exuberance about polyamory as they do from the beginning. There are some people who are ecstatic about the idea and don't find the reality is what they expected. It's not necessarily a bad sign if you're unsure before you try polyamory. But sometimes if you're unsure of whether it's for you, you can end up staying in situations that aren't fantastic for you to prove to yourself or others that you can 'do polyamory'.

Polyamory shouldn't be an emotional obstacle course for you to complete. You're not required to go through a certain amount of pain and discomfort in order to prove or disprove something. There is a huge difference between sitting within discomfort that might come with a big change in how you decide to live your life, especially if you have no models to follow, and forcing yourself into situations that will cause you emotional pain and give you absolutely no benefit in return.

Sometimes people don't particularly see what they're doing when they are attempting to be what I call an 'emotional gladiator'. In previous chapters we discussed agreements where partners only do sexual things with others when their partner is in the room. Another variation on this agreement is wanting to hear or agreeing to tell every detail about other relationships, sexual interests and sexual feelings to each other. On the surface, this sounds great. Don't people make jokes about how polyamorous people are frequent communicators? The first problem with this is that people don't really consider that it can potentially violate the autonomy and privacy of the other people your partner is dating.

Again, applying the same perspective as we have previously, would it ever be necessary for us to divulge details about what we do with other people to family members, friends or other relatives? In fact, if we had a family member who demanded to know the details of dates we went on, we might consider that crossing the line and potentially abusive. Very rarely in the situations where there is an agreement to share all details do I see people asking for the consent of the other person to share details.

Even if the third party consents to sharing details, the idea behind it seems to be like yanking off of a bandage – some type of exposure therapy where if you can listen and sit through the details then it proves you can 'do polyamory'. But there isn't a special prize for being able to hear the most details of your partner with others without breaking a sweat or crying. You aren't better at polyamory just by virtue of not being bothered by listening to details or seeing your partner with other people.

Some people might be genuinely bothered by hearing details of their partner with others. Some people might find that sexy or interesting. Some people, like myself, are not really bothered by it either way. It might occasionally make me feel a bit of a panic, especially on a bad day and I'm generally as uninterested in hearing details with my partners as I am with friends. It's a little bit more convenient in life not to have something that might upset you, but it doesn't necessarily make you a worse person or 'bad at polyamory' to be on the end of the spectrum that might struggle with the details.

Making the shift to polyamory when you've grown up in a mono-centric society and especially if you do not know any other polyamorous people or haven't been shown any other script of doing polyamory before is already taxing enough for the nervous system to adjust to. It already gives you enough to panic and worry about – why force yourself into a situation where you will be even more stressed out? Forcing yourself to hear the ins and outs of a situation, whether to inoculate you against jealousy or to prove something to someone, isn't doing you any favours. It's the equivalent of deciding to move and refusing to use a hand truck or a moving van because you want to prove that you can do everything yourself.

Being an emotional gladiator might seem to be useful in a lot of situations. Your partner may not have to worry that they might say something about another partner that could upset you. Maybe it would be easier if we could all never have any emotional reaction to anything ever – but it's not realistic or fair to expect of yourself and you're not going to magically become more emotionally resilient by forcing yourself to through as much pain as humanly possible.

There is an element of sitting in discomfort when it comes to polyamory. You will probably experience a lot of worry and panic. It's not about avoiding all discomfort, because that's impossible. And I won't pretend that it's easy to tell the difference if you know that you have a habit of struggling to enact boundaries and feeling confident in them. Communication with your partner and the ability to change your mind on things is what makes things like this easier to cope with.

If you have the type of relationship where you've hardly ever complained or been honest with your partner about issues that you've had within the relationship, this might be incredibly difficult to learn to do. Personally, I always believed that conflict was some kind of sign of an oncoming breakup. Having petty arguments about things stressed me out, not just because of the argument but because I thought it was a 'sign' of breaking up. Slowly, I had to learn to deal with conflict, but also let conflict go and not assume that our conflicts meant the end of our relationship.

Either way, whether you tend to clam up and try to put up with everything or force yourself to hear everything, remember that this is a relationship, not an obstacle course. There will absolutely be some emotional resiliency to build, but none of that is solved by forcing yourself to do everything alone. Sometimes a polyamory-friendly therapist might be an important part of learning that balance, but you don't have to prove anything to anyone. And, as I've said in my columns, it's unlikely you actually want your tombstone to say, 'Here Lies [Name]. They could put up with so much before they cracked.'

When comparisons are apt

While it's unwise to try and compare yourself to other partners, a comparison that can be apt is the way your partner treats or prioritizes you in comparison to other partners. While no two relationships are identical and we can often have different energy levels for different people depending on what's going on in our lives, it's still important for you to pay attention to whether you feel fairly treated in comparison.

This isn't to say that your focus and energy has to necessarily be balanced between all partners equally – there might be reasons for focusing on one person and things may shift as time and other events change in our lives. This is pretty normal even within our friendships. If one of our friends is going through a breakup or a death and asks for our support, we might shift our focus from others to that friend. That's to be expected in certain situations.

However, it's quite typical when dating someone new to find yourself wanting to focus on them more and spend time with them more, 'new relationship energy' is the term which is usually given to this phenomenon. Sometimes, especially if it's your first experience with polyamory, you can feel intimidated by your partner's excitement about a new relationship. It can feel like at the time when you need your partner the most, they are not available to provide you with the support that you really need.

While I do think that it's important to keep in mind all of your relationships when you enter a new one, just like you shouldn't blank and ignore your friends just because you're dating someone new, I also think that if people are aware that this is a very common thing for most people to experience, then they might not take their partner getting swept up in new relationship energy so personally or at least they'll feel a little bit calmer if it does happen.

However, whenever you do have a situation where your partner is focusing more attention on others and you feel like your relationship is suffering as a result, it's worth trying your best not to focus on the other person and your partner's relationship with them and instead focus on what is lacking from your relationship with your partner. If you are like I was and struggle to actually speak out when you're not feeling good, then you can feel conflicted about being too anxious to mention what's lacking until you see it in their other relationships but it's better to bring it up later than never.

Leading the conversation with your needs instead of leading with what your partner is doing with others will help focus it on what it should focus on. Picking that apart may require someone else's help but, eventually, you'll become sufficiently familiar with your responses to identify when you're making a comparison that is unhelpful and when you're making one that causes you to re-examine the relationship you have with your partner.

It's okay to do a bit of comparison when it applies to noticing that you're not getting something that you need or want.

PROS AND CONS

As with any decision you make in your life that could potentially alter its course, it's worth continuously checking in with yourself to make sure that the benefits of what you've decided to do outweigh the negatives. What you consider a benefit and a negative might also shift as time goes on, but it's definitely worth really considering your options and remembering that there is always an option to change your mind later on without shame.

Some of the trickier aspects of this might be difficult to pick apart. If we all judged our ability to 'do monogamy' by our very first monogamous relationships, we might have assumed we were incapable of doing it – and that may very well be the experience some people have. The difficulty with something like polyamory versus another lifestyle decision such as moving to the country instead of living in a city is that, when you're talking about a relationship, there's so much within that that's out of your control. It's comfortable to believe that we can study human psychology, relationships and communication, and then we can work our way out of any relationship problem that presents itself, but that's not really the case.

Continuously checking in with yourself is an important part of making a large change but, over time, with the exposure that you have to the polyam community, it can feel like going back to monogamy is less of a change and more of a personal failure.

The validity of monogamy
I spoke in previous chapters about the way polyamory can feel freeing and I don't doubt that a lot of people really struggle within the confines that society places on monogamy. There

are a lot of power structures involved in what messages we're given about the specific type of monogamy we should practise. A lot of relationships that call into question the 'naturalness' of cisgender heterosexual monogamy are frequently condemned and ostracized precisely because they call these assumptions into question and therefore threaten the power that these relationships have in society. When we get out of those narratives, it can feel incredibly freeing, especially if we have been condemned in all sorts of ways for just being ourselves.

Learning about polyamory might be the first time that someone is exposed to anything challenging these cultural influences, so when they decide to try polyamory, it may be specifically freeing because of that challenge. They can then look back on monogamy with the lens of all of the specific things they were told about attached to it and carry resentment for it. Some articles about polyamory, even if they don't explicitly state that monogamy is a negative thing, imply it heavily through a discussion about how polyamory has freed them or taught them something that monogamy hasn't. And while I don't doubt their personal individual experience, I think that it's also easy to forget that a lot of what has been sitting on them isn't monogamy itself.

Perhaps it's specifically due to my thyroid issues and the way that social interaction drains me, but I can absolutely understand the choice to do monogamy simply because you cannot be bothered to date more than one person at a time. One of the first major articles I wrote about polyamory was about how the practice of it is a privilege. While I no longer feel like 'privilege' is a useful framework to apply to every situation, I do feel like many aspects of dating multiple people create obstacles for people who do not have time, money and energy to spare.

Specifically, as a disabled person, I felt an expectation to date loads more than I was and ran myself ragged by forcing myself into multiple social situations that weren't useful or helpful for me. So, I can absolutely understand why and how one can ethically choose to date one person at a time and agree to that with one partner and it not be about controlling your partner's behaviour or limiting their ability to develop other relationships.

Monogamy itself is purely the practice of maintaining one specified romantic relationship at a time. Just as polyamory doesn't come with a degree in relationship dynamics or a commitment to honesty or integrity, monogamy doesn't come with an agreement that possessive jealousy is a positive sign of love or a belief that you ought to be everything for one partner. We shouldn't see an identity or a choice as an endorsement of the roles our society enforces based on that identity.

It's important when reading some of the information about polyamory not just to be aware of the rose-tinted view that often comes with it, but also to spot where there is an assumption that monogamy *can't* have the positive aspects that people claim are exclusive to polyamory. Be aware of the way you might feel a pressure to 'do polyamory' well because going back to monogamy seems to be going back in time, going back in evolution, something to be ashamed of, or going back to a place that endorses possessive jealousy, unequal relationship dynamics and a lack of communication.

There are too many letters I've received (and one is too many but there have been a lot) from people who are specifically being pressured to try polyamory by someone who 'doesn't believe in monogamy' or who has adopted the rhetoric of articles they've read and weaponized it to criticize their partner's preferred way of doing relationships. Their arguments always boil down to an assumption that monogamy is inherently unethical and the clear logical choice is polyamory.

Monogamy is a valid choice and choosing it doesn't make you insecure, archaic or bad. In some cases, the other partner who is adding the pressure isn't intending to make their partner feel like there's something wrong with them for wanting to be monogamous, but they have an earnest wish to try it and feel like a logical, social argument is the best way to convince their partner. They might be excited that they've discovered an aspect of themself isn't as abnormal as they have been encouraged to think. They might also feel resentful about how they've been taught their whole lives that monogamy is the only suitable or meaningful option.

Again, it's hard for me to tell any individual if polyamory is right for them or if in any given moment it's 'worth it', but one thing that can help you weigh up the pros and the cons is if you don't see choosing monogamy as an inherent failure or a sign that you're unable to hack it. In your first experiences within many polyamory communities, you might see anything from articles that casually suggest things like possessiveness is encouraged and welcomed in all monogamy, to people outright saying that monogamous people are pitiful or less evolved. It can be hard if you feel welcomed into a new club of people who are promising you a new level of happiness not to want to kick monogamy when it's down, so to speak, especially if you feel like you previously had no choice but monogamy.

Unfortunately, the truth is that there may be people who judge you if you decide polyamory isn't for you but there is only so much that you can control about that. For me, I found it difficult to be part of communities where polyamory seemed to be the biggest and most interesting thing anyone had to discuss about themselves. Polyamory is something that I do, but I don't see it as so integral to my identity that I need to form bonds with other people who do it in order to feel safe. When you first try polyamory, it may be that it's comforting to have a community behind you that you can go through those experiences with, but the people in the community have to be willing to actually talk about their struggles.

Seeing monogamy as a valid choice that isn't inherently tied to any social convention about how to communicate or arrange your life is an important part of being able to not only decide what works for you best, but also not put so much pressure on yourself to prove your polyamory by maintaining as many relationships as possible or feeling insecure if you're only dating one person, or dating no one. Make sure you're aware of the way you and others around you can create a situation where the decision to be monogamous or feeling you are inherently monogamous is coupled with any type of shame.

Relationship anarchy and labels

While I was initially confused and not particularly wowed by the term 'relationship anarchy', as I've developed a better understanding of concepts of anarchism, it's also led me to a better understanding of what relationship anarchy should and does mean. I would definitely invite people to examine Black anarchist readings and understand what anti-hierarchical processes actually mean before applying them to relationships.

I once felt like the concept of relationship anarchy didn't make sense to me as a disabled person because, especially as I age, I will need more active assistance in my life, literally to go about my day-to-day business. From what I have heard about other disabled people's experiences, I will not necessarily be able to rely on the people around me to help me access what I will need to access in order to live.

Given the way mono-centric society typically works, it's understandable that I would feel like my only options for people I can trust are romantic partners, especially as I don't have access to a circle of support through my family.

While a lot of my thoughts about relationship anarchy progressed because of how I learned about anarchy in general, living through Brexit as well as the COVID-19 pandemic as an immunocompromised person who relied on medication to live also made me question some of the assumptions I had about how my hierarchy might keep me safe or protect me.

When one of my life-sustaining medications was put on a list of medicines that might be affected by Brexit, I really began to question my assumption that money alone was the only incentive needed to encourage the production of the medicine that helped me stay alive. While the government wasn't even instituting proper lockdown measures, I was shielding at home and, as the online grocery store slots became fully booked because of the rush, mutual aid groups were the only way I was able to get food without putting myself at enormous risk. In that situation, it wasn't romantic partners who could help protect me. Erecting a small hierarchy could not necessarily keep me safe in all situations.

Mutual aid is one of the key concepts of anarchism and it's specifically about creating networks of solidarity, not charity. It's about helping each other, rather than creating a system where one person helps from on high. In reading more about anarchism as a concept, I realized that the reason no one could ensure me a picture-perfect future where I would get all of my needs met as a disabled person was because anarchism wasn't about one person deciding what was best for all, or a state deciding what was best for all, but about everyone being able to have an equal voice. I had clung to the acceptance that the only way to do things was the way we were doing things, because I had my medicine at least, but that was never a guarantee. I had just been suckered into believing it was.

When I applied this framework to relationships, I saw a lot of parallels. Monogamy isn't an inherently safer approach; it's just backed up by systems and a seemingly longer tradition. Venturing out into what feels like a new way of doing things is scary, but that doesn't mean it's less safe. Putting a confirmed hierarchy in place also felt a lot safer for me, especially as a disabled person, and stating that I wouldn't have a hierarchy felt like I would have no one to help me when I needed it, but the assumption my romantic partners would be capable of helping me in the ways I needed was just that – an assumption.

While I'm not going to claim to be an 'expert' on relationship anarchy in the same way I don't claim to be an 'expert' in any relationship style, I feel like the way that the concept is communicated is confusing and leads people towards misunderstanding and therefore misusing the concept. As I've learned through anarchist reading, anarchism is not chaos. It doesn't mean society will not have a structure or there will be no processes or anything else put in place. It just means that those processes will be decided by people on a communal level rather than dictated by the state.

Similarly, relationship anarchy, as I understand it, is not about not having any structure, boundaries or ideas of how you might spend your time between relationships, but instead it's about those decisions not being dictated to you by cultural norms and attitudes – or other people. I've been hesitant to describe myself as polyamorous because of the experiences I've had in the polyamory community and wanting to distance myself from that concept, but I'm now reaching a point where I may prefer non-monogamous or relationship anarchist simply because I don't want how I choose to have relationships to be dictated to me – either in the assumption I should only have one or only have multiple and that they should look a certain way or be a certain thing.

I feel like it could be theoretically possible for someone who is a relationship anarchist to look 'monogamous' in their practice of how they do relationships, especially as their energies and ability to devote time to others shift and wane. Just as I don't always feel like sexuality labels can be useful to me, I often feel like the polyamorous/monogamous binary isn't necessarily useful for me and relationship anarchy will often give me the freedom to choose how I want to go about things without being strictly defined in any specific way.

The mistake I also made in my first judgements and observations of relationship anarchy was that it allowed people to basically shy away from emotional commitment to their partners in the same way that my assumption of anarchism was that it allowed people to 'get away' with committing crime or being cruel. While I did see people who claimed to practise relationship anarchy using the practice itself as a way of refusing to support a partner when they needed it, I realized that the practice itself should instead involve the opposite – actively choosing and communicating your needs and deciding what you want rather than letting that be dictated by others.

It's possible in trying polyamory you might find the labels particularly challenging or unhelpful in how you choose to structure your life and relationships. I'm not here to sell you on a specific anti-hierarchical approach. I hesitate to judge the health or benefit of a relationship based on hierarchy alone. However, it might be worth exploring what assumptions you've made about how you value different relationships and interactions. While it might be *possible* to practise monogamy in a way that challenges hierarchies, you might find it difficult to find monogamous people who are necessarily interested in challenging some of the ideas they've learned.

While I'm no longer a fan of necessarily dictating a clear hierarchy in how I'm going to spend my time and energy, I still make an effort to make sure that I'm clear about what I want, if and when things shift. If you're deciding on what a pro or a con is for what you're practising, consider that it might not be a non-monogamous practice that is the issue for you, but the way that you might feel expected to define or practise it.

PERSPECTIVE CHALLENGE

It can be easy to lose sight of the larger picture when you're in the middle of a situation or find a way to reframe your perspective if you're in the midst of a lot of emotions and fears. This challenge could be done when you're trying to make sense of a situation or to run through scenarios where you might anticipate problems.

Ask yourself these questions but feel free to include or remove individuals involved as they apply to your situation:

How differently would you feel if one of the individuals involved in this situation was a friend whom you are not romantically or sexually involved with?

. . . .

. . . .

. . . .

. . . .

. . . .

How differently would you feel if all the individuals involved were non-romantic, platonic friends?

. . . .

. . . .

. . . .

. . . .

. . . .

How differently would you feel if one or all the individuals involved in this scenario were a family member or if the situations involved were about family rather than romantic or sexual dynamics?

. . . .

. . . .

. . . .

. . . .

. . . .

What do you think your partner(s) is feeling in this situation? What pressures do you think they are experiencing? What pressures are you experiencing that you feel your partner(s) may not be?

. . . .

. . . .

. . . .

. . . .

. . . .

What do you think anyone else involved in this situation is feeling? What pressures do you think they are experiencing? What pressures are you experiencing that you feel others may not be?

. . . .

. . . .

. . . .

. . . .

. . . .

What is the worst-case scenario of this situation? What is the best-case scenario?

. . . .

. . . .

. . . .

. . . .

. . . .

If the worst-case scenario were to occur, what would your next step be and how would you continue to support yourself?

. . . .

. . . .

. . . .

. . . .

. . . .

While the Perspective Challenge isn't meant to solve everything about a situation, I personally find that I can struggle to remember that not everyone has all the information about my personal situation that I have and, likewise, I do not have all of the information that they have. In many situations, we can operate based on assumptions we have about the other person rather than what is actually known.

Once you have written out what you know about the situation, you may wish to confer with a therapist or with your partner(s) or any of the people involved in the situation to see if you can come to an understanding, but it's worth keeping in mind that if someone is not coming into the situation in good faith and doesn't desire to make peace out of it, there isn't much about that you can change.

RELATIONSHIP CHECK-UP

While these discussions don't have to be highly formalized or official, it's worth checking in with your partner every once in a while to make sure you're on the same page when it comes to your relationship and your life goals. The frequency with which you decide to do this can be weekly, monthly, quarterly or yearly and this can change depending on changes of circumstances within your life or the life of any of your partners.

You have the option of reviewing these on your own and then coming together with a partner to review these together.

Have your original desires for how you do relationships changed since your last check-up?

. . . .

. . . .

. . . .

. . . .

What has been bringing you more stress recently?

. . . .

. . . .

. . . .

. . . .

What has been helping you overcome stress recently?

. . . .

. . . .

. . . .

. . . .

How has your relationship helped contribute positively to your life recently?

. . . .

. . . .

. . . .

. . . .

What in your relationship has been more challenging recently?

. . . .

. . . .

. . . .

. . . .

Are there steps you can take together to change or improve anything?

. . . .

. . . .

. . . .

. . . .

If you took some steps since the last check-in to change, how has that worked out?

. . . .

. . . .

. . . .

. . . .

What do you foresee impacting both yourself and your relationships in the near future?

. . . .

. . . .

. . . .

. . . .

Can you think of five things that make you grateful for your partners?

. . . .

. . . .

. . . .

. . . .

What do you feel your relationships have brought to your life?

. . . .

. . . .

. . . .

. . . .

What, if anything, do you feel is overall missing in your life?

. . . .

. . . .

. . . .

. . . .

ANXIETY TOOLKIT

Everyone will have a different experience with anxiety and the reasons behind it. There are only so many self-help books you can read, quizzes you can take and exercises you can do if you're in a relationship that is constantly causing you anxiety. Just because you can cope with anxiety doesn't mean you should continuously subject yourself to situations that cause it if you can avoid it.

This toolkit is what I use to help me walk through my anxiety and learn how to understand it, cope with it and take any steps needed to address it. It doesn't mean you will never experience anxiety again, but you may find that once you feel more capable of coping with anxiety, you're able to get to a place where you don't begin to spiral as easily.

It's always worth considering speaking to a polyamory-friendly relationship therapist to help you work through recurring anxiety issues. It can be easy, especially if you've been through any kind of childhood trauma, to believe that everything is your fault and many modern polyamory advice websites teach you how to self-gaslight and think every problem is yours to fix and handle. If you are experiencing recurring anxiety, it may be worth it to walk through your problems with a therapist, who may be able to help you get a better picture.

Furthermore, it's worth noting that this is mainly for anxiety that seems to come out of nowhere. If you are changing jobs, experiencing a bereavement, moving or doing another major life shift, it's normal for you to feel anxiety. It may still help you to work through the toolkit but those will have different causes than these.

Step 1: Identifying the source of the anxiety

What is the problem your anxiety is presenting?

. . . .

. . . .

. . . .

. . . .

Is this a problem that you feel you've had before in other relationships?

. . . .

. . . .

. . . .

. . . .

Is this a recurring fear or problem or connected to another problem?

. . . .

. . . .

. . . .

. . . .

The point of this section is to help you figure out if this is a recurring issue throughout your life. A lot of our anxiety gets activated or peeks through when there is a situation that feels life threatening, even if it may not be.

Step 2: Identifying the motive of the anxiety

If you had unlimited power, what would you be able to do to address this anxiety?

. . . .

. . . .

. . . .

. . . .

What about this situation is under your immediate control?

. . . .

. . . .

. . . .

. . . .

What about this situation is *not* under your immediate control?

. . . .

. . . .

. . . .

. . . .

If you could instantly solve this problem, how would it make you feel?

. . . .

. . . .

. . . .

. . . .

What need would instantly curing this anxiety meet?

. . . .

. . . .

. . . .

. . . .

Identifying what you could do if you could instantly cure this anxiety can often lead you to its motive. A lot of anxiety boils down to survival, but it's helpful to figure out what it's trying to protect and whether there is any aspect of the situation you can actually control.

Step 3: Enacting compassion on yourself

How can solving your problem help you survive?

. . . .

. . . .

. . . .

. . . .

If you can think back to some of the times you've had in your life where similar fears have come up, what did you have in the way of support?

. . . .

. . . .

. . . .

. . . .

If you could not solve this problem yourself, who would have supported you in solving this problem?

. . . .

. . . .

. . . .

. . . .

If the worst were to happen and your anxiety were to come true, what would happen to you afterwards?

. . . .

. . . .

. . . .

. . . .

Can you see what you're trying to protect yourself from when you imagine the worst?

. . . .

. . . .

. . . .

. . . .

The point of this section is to help you feel more compassion towards yourself. Our anxieties sometimes are trying to protect us from the worst things that can happen to us. But unfortunately, we can't assume we have control over that without also blaming ourselves for situations in our past where we were in danger or got hurt. Learning how to have compassion for my anxiety and what it was trying to do helped me cope with it.

Step 4: Sitting within discomfort

What situations have you been through before that you have overcome?

. . . .

. . . .

. . . .

. . . .

In what ways will you be able to take care of yourself in situations where you're in distress? How have you taken care of yourself in the past?

. . . .

. . . .

. . . .

. . . .

Which friends, family members, partners and others do you feel you can rely on during difficult times?

. . . .

. . . .

. . . .

. . . .

What would you say to a friend who is going through the same thing you currently are?

. . . .

. . . .

. . . .

. . . .

What can you do to take care of yourself in the current moment?

. . . .

. . . .

. . . .

. . . .

What basic needs can you address now that you may not have addressed yet such as eating, drinking, bathing, movement, social interaction or rest?

. . . .

. . . .

. . . .

. . . .

How has this incident of anxiety been different to other incidents?

. . . .

. . . .

. . . .

The point of this section is to help you find tools to sit within the discomfort anxiety can bring. Anxiety definitely does have valleys as much as it has peaks and feeling like you can manage the more difficult situations will help you build more tolerance in the future.

Again, if the source of your anxiety is your relationship and you repeatedly see no improvement, it might be worth exploring your situation with a polyamory-friendly therapist, who might be able to help you walk through your options. If polyamory is not something that you want to do, you will continuously have anxiety and there is only so much you're going to be able to do to counteract that.

UNHELPFUL ASSUMPTIONS

Our society encourages us to believe a lot of things about relationships that create expectations that often our partners can't or shouldn't meet. Even within monogamous relationships, these assumptions can create conflict where there need not be any. Below is a list of assumptions that many may have picked up from a variety of sources that may not be helpful.

It's not necessarily terrible to believe in some aspects of these assumptions, but it's when you make them into gospel or attempt to hold your partners to them that it can create problems. Feel free to use these as journaling prompts to explore how you came by this assumption and the impact it's had within your relationships. These can also be discussion topics you can have with partners.

For the purposes of addressing some of the issues that you may come across in polyamory, I will also include some of the assumptions I find unhelpful within polyamory advice and communities.

You should only ever be attracted to your partners sexually.

It's not unusual for people, even monogamous ones, to experience attraction to others romantically, aesthetically, sexually and more. Expecting your partner to only ever be attracted to you is unrealistic.

Being friends with exes means you haven't gotten over them.

Many people maintain positive relationships with their ex-partners all the time without there being any interest in a relationship. Assuming your partner has not 'gotten over' their ex demonstrates a lack of trust in them, which will inevitably lead to problems later on. You should begin from a place of trust in relationships or be working towards that.

If you and your partner are truly compatible, you won't ever have conflict.

Conflict is an inevitable part of *all* relationships and can often help bring friends, families, lovers and communities closer. Environments that don't allow for any conflict become eggshell pits that agitate our nervous systems more over time. Dealing with conflict is difficult, but necessary to do.

You should never go to bed angry, no matter how tired you are.

Sometimes being tired makes it harder for us to communicate effectively. As uncomfortable as it might be, going to bed might be what you need to do to work out a conflict.

It's important to share all your partner's hobbies and activities.

Some partners get together because they share hobbies and activities, but it's not reasonable to expect your partner to be involved in every single activity that you do. Just as it's not reasonable to expect your friends to be interested in all the same things that you're interested in.

If your partner has a close friend, that's a sign the friend is secretly trying to steal your partner.

No one can 'steal' your partner. Your partner can choose, either through lacking their own boundaries and autonomy or through their own decision-making process, to be with someone else instead of you or 'replace' you in a way. Removing the agency from your partner and assigning it to a friend makes sense because it's easier for you to direct your fears onto a person you don't love.

But your partner is the one that makes that decision. And having a close friend doesn't mean that your partner is out to replace you. We need all types of relationships in our lives. If your partner treats you as if you are replaceable, that is an issue with your partner and not the friend they are with.

Someone who is better than you can steal your partner from you.

Again, no one can 'steal' your partner from you. I won't pretend there isn't inherently a risk as there is within all relationships that your relationship could end. But that doesn't necessarily mean you can control it.

Thoughts like this make you feel more empowered because you feel like you can 'win' your partner by being the 'best', which is something you can control. Unfortunately, outside of treating your partner and yourself well, there is nothing you can do to prevent them from falling out of love with you.

Your partner has chosen you because you are the best person they could find.

This might be true of your partner, particularly if they are buying into other toxic ideas about relationships. But this isn't something you can control either. If your partner chooses to see you as a replaceable feature in their life or uses you, you can't control that. You can only control how long you're willing to put up with it.

Relationships are only valuable and important if they are long term.

It sucks to break up, without a doubt. It's usually painful and can involve a change in our day-to-day lives that is a struggle. But that doesn't mean we should always have to aim for a long-term relationship or that only long-term relationships are worthy or valuable.

Relationships can be valuable regardless of their length. And when we assume that only long-term relationships are valuable, we feel like an extra failure when they end. But relationships of all kinds have value.

All relationships must include sex.

Asexual people exist and they may very well want to have a romantic relationship that does not include sex. Sex drives and the amount of sex had in a relationship may change over time. What's important is whether it's communicated with each other, boundaries are agreed upon and if it's working for everyone involved.

Your partner not wanting to have sex with you is because something is wrong with you.

Sex drives can vary over time. Your partner not wanting to have sex with you doesn't mean you've done anything wrong. Being rejected is difficult and it's understandable to feel some emotions about that, maybe even feel frustrated. Many people struggle with rejection even if they feel otherwise safe in a relationship. If your partner explicitly says they are withholding sex as a means of punishment, this is something that you'll need to address. While your partner isn't obligated to have sex with you, they shouldn't be using it as a way to control you.

You should try to control your partner's emotions by behaving in ways you know they will like.

While we all want our partners to be happy and want to try and improve their lives, there is only so much we can control about our partner's emotions. Believing that you can control your partner's feelings or attempting to isn't always done from a place of malice or manipulation – sometimes we just want to prevent ourselves from getting hurt.

But it's important not only to avoid trying to manipulate situations in ways that will benefit us, but also to be honest with our partners about how we feel instead of putting on a brave face just for them.

Not remembering important dates means your partner doesn't care.

Not everyone is good at remembering dates. While we can make an effort to remind ourselves, just because a date is not remembered doesn't mean your partner doesn't care. It's important to have a discussion with your partner about key dates and what you feel is important to do on those dates so you don't get disappointed.

Not noticing a change in your appearance means your partner doesn't care.

Some people can notice small changes in their partner's appearances, but others may find it difficult to do so due to their neurology and the way their brain works. Not noticing isn't a sign that your partner doesn't care about what you do for them.

Even if it's nice for someone to notice something without you pointing it out, having the expectation that they will do so might be unfair to them, especially if you take it personally if they don't.

It's a bad sign if your partner needs time alone.

Some people need more alone time than others and sometimes during a conflict people need time alone to be able to reflect and get their words together. Needing time alone or space doesn't necessarily mean someone is angry and it's not an immediate bad sign.

I know in the past if my partner wasn't willing to speak with me when I needed them to, my anxiety would cause me to jump to the worst possible conclusions. But it was unfair of me to expect any of my partners to be immediately ready for the conversation I wanted to have. Sometimes people need time alone, and that's that.

Your partner should always come to you first if they want to have any sexual interaction, even with themselves.

Sexual relationships, including the one we have with ourselves, are different. There are different things we get from these experiences that we don't necessarily get through others. I constantly struggle with the idea that I'm not 'useful' enough if my partner doesn't come to me first for a sexual need because I've had a lot of relationships where I only got the love I needed by being useful.

I tend to feel that if I'm not 'useful' to someone, I will be discarded for someone who is more 'useful'. Putting this kind of pressure on me wouldn't be fair in any relationship and it's also not fair for anyone I date to feel that way. Even though logically now I understand how to manage it, the feeling still pops up.

Your partner has a right to criticize your looks and appearance.

People have preferences and it's understandable to want to be appealing to your partners. It's one thing if you decide that you want to cut your hair in a certain way or wear something that you know your partner would like, but it is never a good sign when a partner has something pejorative and negative to say about your appearance, especially if they are equating it to your overall worth as a human being.

Your partner should also never be encouraging you to threaten your health or wellbeing purely for the purposes of looking more appealing to them.

Relationships should be hard.

Relationships take work and there are sometimes low parts of relationships that create a lot of conflict and anxiety in our life, but, overall, the net benefit you gain from a relationship should be more than its negatives. While there might be times when we are supporting our partners a bit more than they are supporting us, such as when they have a crisis in their lives, that support should feel potentially reciprocal.

It can be hard to let go of a relationship where you feel needed, especially if you don't have much experience of feeling wanted in your life, but it's important to make sure that you feel just as supported, as you are supportive.

An end to a relationship represents a failure on one or both sides.

Relationships end for a variety of reasons and it doesn't necessarily represent failure on your or your partner's side. Two people can be great communicators who are very in touch with their needs who are just incompatible. Sometimes relationships don't work out despite both sides trying to make it work.

While it's understandable to mourn the loss of a relationship or feel fear about your life changing, it's important to remember to avoid blaming yourself. After you have had the chance to mourn and heal, you may identify actions that you took that you wouldn't take now, but you can do that without blaming yourself in a way that encourages you to feel ashamed or attack yourself.

Talking about sex and relationships makes you a clingy or needy person.

Too many films romanticize the idea of a relationship where everything just magically fits and works out without discussions or awkwardness. A lot of people assume that asking for what they want will make them a less enticing partner and, while it might be true that having absolutely no needs whatsoever might make you a very easy person to date, it's not a realistic expectation to have for yourself. You can't change your needs and you shouldn't.

For some people, you might be someone they call 'needy' but you could just as easily see it as them being unable to meet your needs. It's all relative. Just be honest about what you need and let the chips fall where they may.

Friendships mean less than romantic relationships.

While it's up to individuals to define how they deal with relationships, the assumption that friendships are less meaningful than romantic relationships doesn't necessarily hold true for most people's experiences. Romance is *different* to friendship, just like familial relationships are *different* to romance, but it doesn't mean we value our partners inherently more than family members or vice versa. Different relationships are different and have different impacts on our life.

If your relationship is a good one, it should be able to conquer any depression or anxiety.

Despite our culture teaching us that 'love conquers all', mental health isn't something that can be solved by relationships in all cases. While being in a healthy, reciprocal relationship can balance out our nervous systems and relieve stress, it's not necessarily going to solve underlying mental health issues, which may be more complex and difficult to treat. You should never make it your responsibility to cure or fix another person as a lot of that is determined by factors out of your control.

A partner who expresses a high level of love and infatuation within the first few weeks of meeting you is just being sweet and caring.

While it can feel flattering to have someone so interested in you at the beginning of your relationship or even dating someone, sometimes an outpouring of infatuation can lead to an unhappy place later on. It is worth considering whether this might be a case of love-bombing.

Remember that anyone who is worth keeping around would be more than happy to respect your boundaries and take their time getting to know you. Our cultural narrative sometimes excuses possessive and controlling behaviour because someone's love is so strong, but realistically, someone who loves you is someone who respects your boundaries and doesn't want you to feel uncomfortable.

You have a right to go through your partner's phone if they provide you with the password.

Even if partners grant your permission to go through their phone, when you get to a point where you cannot trust your partner and feel like you have to go through their private information, violating not only their privacy but the privacy of the people they are speaking to, you have already reached a crisis point in your relationship that cannot be helped by going through someone's phone.

You don't have an inherent right to violate anyone's privacy, even if you've been in a relationship with someone for a long time and even if they have a history of cheating. Privacy is privacy. While I don't shame people for resorting to this if they feel like they have no other option, you should generally be honest about violating someone else's privacy if you have.

*If your partner **really** loved you, they would stop doing...*

This one can be tricky because it's easy to argue that if your partner cares and loves for you, they will respect your boundaries and treat you with respect, but sometimes things can get a little bit more complex. Even as this type of a rule might help you figure out when you're not being treated well, it could be used by others to manipulate you into doing something to prove your love for them.

Even if someone wants to encourage you to do something small like take out the trash or picking up more after yourself, saying you should be doing it out of love rather than just mutual respect and being a good roommate, as valid as the request may be, doesn't speak particularly well to the motivations of the person asking. If you feel like you have to constantly prove how much you're worth to someone, that may not be a good sign.

Experiencing jealousy means you have poor self esteem.

Jealousy can be an understandable reaction that doesn't have any-thing to do with an individual's self-esteem. Having jealousy is a normal and natural part of living, especially if you're in a relationship that isn't meeting your needs.

Don't assume that being jealous means you have failed or that there is something wrong with you. While sometimes jealousy can be triggered by some of our assumptions of what we've learned within mono-centric culture, it's not always the case.

Having an emotional reaction to a situation is an attempt to control your partner.

Too many polyamory advice articles make it seem like the only way to be 'good at' polyamory is not to have any emotional reaction to anything your partner does and reach a Vulcan-like state of complete detachment. Furthermore, when boundaries are not clearly defined, if your partner does have an emotional reaction to something you do, it can be easy to feel like your only choice is to change your behaviour in order to 'fix' it.

Too often people are not able to sit with the fact that they may be causing their partner discomfort and decide to cancel dates, close relationships or not even date at all to avoid their partner being upset, only to then feel controlled by their partner's emotional reactions. This is somewhat understandable, especially if you have a history of abuse where a partner was violent or used explosive reactions to underhandedly control your behaviour.

However, just because you might *feel* controlled by the fact that your partner is upset doesn't mean your partner is *intentionally* attempting to control you, and it's important to see the distinction. People might have emotional reactions to things and that doesn't always mean they are trying to control you.

Having negative feelings about your partner dating others means you're bad at polyamory.

Negative feelings are as inevitable in polyamory as they are in monogamy. It's unrealistic to expect you never to have any specific issues with your partner dating others when you have been raised within a mono-centric culture that has given you messages your entire life about how love should work.

It's also unrealistic to expect yourself to always feel secure. You may experience less upset or anxiety as you establish safety within your relationship and build trust. But, even after years of feeling secure in your romantic relationship, other occurrences outside of it can leave you vulnerable and scared. The feeling of security can wax and wane. Don't always assume that having negative feelings about your partner dating inherently means you're 'bad at' polyamory.

Not getting along with your metamours means you are jealous.

Sometimes people just don't get along. Would we expect our partners to get along with all our friends if we were monogamous? So why is there an expectation that all metamours should get along? People may not mesh with each other well for all sorts of reasons that have nothing to do with jealousy.

Knowing everything about a relationship your partner has is your right.

No one has an inherent right to know everything about your other relationships. You may agree to give certain details to each other, but that doesn't mean that knowing everything is an inherent right that anyone has. It's worth discussing with all parties what you're willing to disclose and discuss about your partnerships before disclosing details.

Closing a relationship will solve all the problems it being open has caused.

While closing a relationship may address some of the immediate concerns people can have, it can't really solve relationship problems. Even if the problem is that your partner is distracted by a new partner and isn't spending time on your relationship if they are not inclined to do that themselves or listen to your concerns, closing the relationship won't fix that.

Conclusion

∞

My hopes are that by the time you've reached the end of this book, you will have not only a clearer perspective on what non-monogamy can offer you, but also some ideas of how you want to go about it. I hope it's given you some validation for some of the anxieties and fears you've had as well as giving you the ability to fight those anxieties. Or, you may have reached the end of this book deciding that polyamory definitely isn't for you, and that's fine too.

If you're not remotely interested in non-monogamy, maybe this book has given you some tips for having better monogamous relationships. The biggest thing I hope anyone can take away from all of this is a more grounded trust in their own intuition, an ability to make decisions from a grounded perspective and an understanding that you are the best person, in fact the *only* person, who can effectively understand all aspects of your own feelings.

The only person who can tell you for sure if non-monogamy is for you is *you*.

I am not a guru. I am not an expert. That might be an odd thing to read in a self-help book because so many of these books, especially within polyamory, are written from the standpoint of people who, if they don't say they are experts, act like experts. My desire to help and advise other people doesn't come from the place of being all-knowing or never making a mistake. In fact, the mistakes I've made have taught me a lot more than the mistakes

I didn't make. I am sure I will continue to make mistakes and learn from them. My desire to help has never been top-down but side-to-side in solidarity. Its intended purpose is mutual aid.

I'd also like to recognize that my perspective, while it may include some things not common in many polyamory advice perspectives, still comes from a place of privilege in many areas. I'm white, my disabilities are quite often 'hidden' from people in many ways and I'm no longer facing the poverty or broke-ness that I did when I was younger. Seek out perspectives of people who face similar struggles if you can.

I ask anyone who has read this book to see me not as an expert on high, but as someone offering another way of looking at the subject that may help them – my writing is not and cannot be universal.

Take what helps and leave the rest.

Bibliography

Bancroft, L. (2003) *Why Does He Do That? Inside the Minds of Angry and Controlling Men*. New York, NY: Berkley Trade.

Gahran, A. (n.d.) 'What is the Relationship Escalator? – Off the Relationship Escalator.' Off the Relationship Escalator. Retrieved on 31 July 2021 from https://offescalator.com/what-escalator.

Gay, R. (2021) 'Why people are so awful online.' *The New York Times*, 19 July. Retrieved on 05 October 2021 from www.nytimes.com/2021/07/17/opinion/culture/social-media-cancel-culture-roxane-gay.html.

Goldberg, W. (2016) 'Whoopi Goldberg wants to make you feel better.' *The New York Times*, 31 August. Retrieved on 1 November 2021 from www.nytimes.com/2016/09/04/magazine/whoopi-goldberg-wants-to-make-you-feel-better.html.

Kassel, G. (2020) 'What to know about vee relationships, the polyamorous structure some people swear by.' *Well+Good*. Retrieved on 5 October 2021 from www.wellandgood.com/vee-relationship-structure.

Morrigan, C. (2019) *Love Without Emergency: I Want This But I Feel Like I'm Going to Die* [E-book].

Nordgren, A. (2006) 'The short instructional manifesto for relationship anarchy.' The Anarchist Library. Retrieved on 5 October 2021 from https://theanarchistlibrary.org/library/andie-nordgren-the-short-instructional-manifesto-for-relationship-anarchy.

Said, E.W. (1995) *Orientalism: Western Concepts of the Orient*. New York, NY: Penguin Books Ltd, p.10.

Sapolsky, R.M. (2004) *Why Zebras Don't Get Ulcers*. New York, NY: St Martin's Press.

Suggested Reading

If you have been within polyamory communities, you will get referred to these two books frequently: *Opening Up* by Tristan Taormino and *The Ethical Slut* by Dossie Easton and Janet Hardy.

While I don't think they are bad books to read, I wanted to frame my suggested reading not just around relationships, but also around trauma, human behaviour, and how we understand others and ourselves, and provide a more rounded list about social issues in general. The first three are more relationship-related and the rest are on a variety of social issues that might be helpful to consider.

Meg-John Barker, *Rewriting the Rules*

Meg-John Barker has written one of the best books about non-monogamy that I have read that I feel applies to a wide variety of people.

Clementine Morrigan, *Love Without Emergency: I Want This But I Feel Like I'm Going to Die*

Clementine does an amazing job of conveying the experience of polyamory for someone who has gone through trauma.

Kevin Patterson, *Love's Not Color Blind: Race and Representation in Polyamorous and Other Alternative Communities*

Anyone seeking to make polyamorous communities a better place for all should read this book.

Lundy Bancroft, *Why Does He Do That?*

I recommend this frequently on my column and podcast. It's essential for understanding abusive mentalities.

Cordelia Fine, *Delusions of Gender*

This will give you a keener understanding of how studies can be influenced by social structures, even as they claim to be objective.

Caroline Dooner, *The Fuck It Diet*

While this is more about relationships with food, it's given me greater insight into my own anxiety and desire for control.

Robert Sapolsky, *Why Zebras Don't Get Ulcers*

A really good exploration of how stress impacts our bodies and how our bodies can experience life-or-death stress levels in non-life-or-death situations.

Sofie Hagen, *Happy Fat*

A book that goes beyond self-love and how societal conceptions of beauty are about more than just self-esteem but also create power structures.

Edward Said, *Orientalism*

One of my first post-graduate readings beyond 'the West' that talks about how cultural portrayals of 'the Orient' affect power dynamics.

Thomas Kuhn, *The Structure of Scientific Revolutions*

A really brilliant challenge to the assumption that scientific progress is always linear and objective.

Ching-In Chen, Jai Dulani and Leah Lakshmi Plepzna-Samarasinha, *The Revolution Starts at Home*

This has some really practical guidance to understanding how social power dynamics impact our interpersonal relationships.

Ian Ford, *A Field Guide to Earthlings*

An amazing book for anyone looking to understand an autistic experience and how difficult it can be to navigate an allistic (non-autistic) world.

Cacilda Jethá and Christopher Ryan, *Sex at Dawn*

Though widely critiqued, I appreciated the way *Sex at Dawn* challenged assumptions we make about archaeological and cultural findings.

Caitlin Doughty, *Smoke Gets in Your Eyes*

While sex is a cultural taboo, so is death. I appreciated the way this book challenged that within me.

Akala, *Natives*

Specifically for UK-based readers or anyone looking to understand more about the UK, this book gives some great historical understandings of class and race in the UK.

Travis Alabanza, *Before I Step Outside [You Love Me]*

Travis brilliantly speaks about their personal experience in this zine as a trans person navigating public spaces in a profound way.

Index